T0234502

OTHER FAST FACTS BOOKS

Fast Facts About PTSD: A Guide for Nurses and Other Health Care Professionals (*Adams*)

Fast Facts for the NEW NURSE PRACTITIONER: What You Really Need to Know in a Nutshell, Second Edition (*Aktan*)

Fast Facts for NURSE PRACTITIONERS: Practice Essentials for Clinical Subspecialties (*Aktan*)

Fast Facts for the ER NURSE: Emergency Department Orientation in a Nutshell, Third Edition (*Buettner*)

Fast Facts About GI AND LIVER DISEASES FOR NURSES: What APRNs Need to Know in a Nutshell (*Chaney*)

Fast Facts for WRITING THE DNP PROJECT: Effective Structure, Content, and Presentation (*Christenbery*)

Fast Facts for the MEDICAL–SURGICAL NURSE: Clinical Orientation in a Nutshell (*Ciocco*)

Fast Facts on COMBATING NURSE BULLYING, INCIVILITY, AND WORKPLACE VIOLENCE: What Nurses Need to Know in a Nutshell (*Ciocco*)

Fast Facts for the NURSE PRECEPTOR: Keys to Providing a Successful Preceptorship in a Nutshell (*Ciocco*)

Fast Facts for the OPERATING ROOM NURSE: An Orientation and Care Guide, Second Edition (*Criscitelli*)

Fast Facts for the ANTEPARTUM AND POSTPARTUM NURSE: A Nursing Orientation and Care Guide in a Nutshell (*Davidson*)

Fast Facts for the NEONATAL NURSE: A Nursing Orientation and Care Guide in a Nutshell (*Davidson*)

Fast Facts Workbook for CARDIAC DYSRHYTHMIAS AND 12-LEAD EKGs (*Desmarais*)

Fast Facts About PRESSURE ULCER CARE FOR NURSES: How to Prevent, Detect, and Resolve Them in a Nutshell (*Dziedzic*)

Fast Facts for the GERONTOLOGY NURSE: A Nursing Care Guide in a Nutshell (*Eliopoulos*)

Fast Facts for the LONG-TERM CARE NURSE: What Nursing Home and Assisted Living Nurses Need to Know in a Nutshell (*Eliopoulos*)

Fast Facts for the CLINICAL NURSE MANAGER: Managing a Changing Workplace in a Nutshell, Second Edition (*Fry*)

Fast Facts for EVIDENCE-BASED PRACTICE IN NURSING: Third Edition (*Godshall*)

Fast Facts for Nurses About HOME INFUSION THERAPY: The Expert's Best Practice Guide in a Nutshell (*Gorski*)

Fast Facts About NURSING AND THE LAW: Law for Nurses in a Nutshell (*Grant, Ballard*)

Fast Facts for the L&D NURSE: Labor & Delivery Orientation in a Nutshell, Second Edition (*Groll*)

Fast Facts for the RADIOLOGY NURSE: An Orientation and Nursing Care Guide, Second Edition (*Grossman*)

Fast Facts in HEALTH INFORMATICS FOR NURSES (*Hardy*)

Fast Facts on ADOLESCENT HEALTH FOR NURSING AND HEALTH PROFESSIONALS: A Care Guide in a Nutshell (*Herrman*)

Fast Facts for the CRITICAL CARE NURSE, Second Edition (*Hewett*)

Fast Facts for the FAITH COMMUNITY NURSE: Implementing FCN/Parish Nursing in a Nutshell (*Hickman*)

Fast Facts for the CARDIAC SURGERY NURSE: Caring for Cardiac Surgery Patients, Third Edition (*Hodge*)

Fast Facts About the NURSING PROFESSION: Historical Perspectives in a Nutshell (*Hunt*)

Fast Facts for the NURSE PSYCHOTHERAPIST: The Process of Becoming (*Jones, Tusaie*)

Fast Facts for the CLINICAL NURSING INSTRUCTOR: Clinical Teaching in a Nutshell, Third Edition (*Kan, Stabler-Haas*)

Fast Facts for the WOUND CARE NURSE: Practical Wound Management in a Nutshell (*Kifer*)

Fast Facts About EKGs FOR NURSES: The Rules of Identifying EKGs in a Nutshell (*Landrum*)

Fast Facts for the TRAVEL NURSE: Travel Nursing in a Nutshell (*Landrum*)

Fast Facts for the SCHOOL NURSE: What You Need to Know, Third Edition (*Loschiavo*)

Fast Facts to LOVING YOUR RESEARCH PROJECT: A Stress-Free Guide for Novice Researchers in Nursing and Healthcare (*Marshall*)

Fast Facts for MANAGING PATIENTS WITH A PSYCHIATRIC DISORDER: What RNs, NPs, and New Psych Nurses Need to Know (*Marshall*)

Forthcoming FAST FACTS Books

Visit www.springerpub.com to order.

FAST FACTS for
DEMENTIA CARE

Carol A. Miller, MSN, RN-BC, has addressed the needs of older adults who have dementia for more than four decades in numerous clinical settings, including hospitals, a geropsychiatric program, long-term care facilities, and community-based programs. She has held clinical positions as a nurse practitioner, geriatric care manager, consultant, administrator, and interprofessional team member. Ms. Miller has served on the professional advisory board of the Alzheimer's Association and is widely recognized as an expert in the care of older adults, with particular expertise in person-centered care for people with dementia.

Ms. Miller has held various faculty positions at the Francis Payne Bolton School of Nursing at Case Western Reserve University and a host of other nursing programs. Her professional publications include *Elder Abuse and Nursing: What Nurses Need to Know and Can Do About It* and eight editions of *Nursing for Wellness in Older Adults*, which has received two *American Journal of Nursing* Book of the Year Awards in gerontology. She has presented at numerous professional organizations and served for 2 years as a spokesperson for a national health education campaign on issues related to caregiving, a role that involved appearances on hundreds of radio and TV programs, including *Good Morning America*.

FAST FACTS for
DEMENTIA CARE

What Nurses Need to Know

Second Edition

Carol A. Miller, MSN, RN-BC

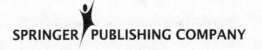

SPRINGER PUBLISHING COMPANY

First Springer Publishing edition: 2012
No part of this publication may be reproduced, stored in a retrieval system, or trans-
mitted in any form or by any means, electronic, mechanical, photocopying, recording,
or otherwise, without the prior permission of Springer Publishing Company, LLC, or
authorization through payment of the appropriate fees to the Copyright Clearance
Center, Inc., 222 Rosewood Drive, Danvers, MA 01923, 978-750-8400, fax 978-646-
8600, info@copyright.com or on the Web at www.copyright.com.

Springer Publishing Company, LLC
11 West 42nd Street, New York, NY 10036
www.springerpub.com
connect.springerpub.com/

Acquisitions Editor: Rachel Landes
Compositor: Amnet Systems

ISBN: 978-0-8261-5171-1
ebook ISBN: 978-0-8261-5181-0
DOI: 10.1891/9780826151810

20 21 22 23 / 5 4 3 2 1

The author and the publisher of this Work have made every effort to use sources believed
to be reliable to provide information that is accurate and compatible with the standards
generally accepted at the time of publication. Because medical science is continually
advancing, our knowledge base continues to expand. Therefore, as new information
becomes available, changes in procedures become necessary. We recommend that the
reader always consult current research and specific institutional policies before performing any clinical procedure or delivering any medication. The author and publisher
shall not be liable for any special, consequential, or exemplary damages resulting, in
whole or in part, from the readers' use of, or reliance on, the information contained in
this book. The publisher has no responsibility for the persistence or accuracy of URLs
for external or third-party Internet websites referred to in this publication and does not
guarantee that any content on such websites is, or will remain, accurate or appropriate.

Library of Congress Cataloging-in-Publication Data

Names: Miller, Carol A., author.
Title: Fast facts for dementia care : what nurses need to know / Carol A. Miller.
Other titles: Fast facts (Springer Publishing Company)
Description: Second edition. | New York : Springer Publishing Company,
    [2021] | Series: Fast facts | Includes bibliographical references and index.
Identifiers: LCCN 2020008105 | ISBN 9780826151711 (paperback) | ISBN
    9780826151810 (ebook)
Subjects: MESH: Dementia—nursing | Geriatric Nursing—methods
Classification: LCC RC521 | NLM WY 152 | DDC 616.8/310231—dc23
LC record available at https://lccn.loc.gov/2020008105

Contact us to receive discount rates on bulk purchases.
We can also customize our books to meet your needs.
For more information please contact: sales@springerpub.com

Publisher's Note: New and used products purchased from third-party sellers are not
guaranteed for quality, authenticity, or access to any included digital components.

Printed in the United States of America.

Contents

Part I DEMENTIA: WHAT IT IS, WHAT IT IS NOT, AND WHAT NURSES CAN DO

Part II PERSON-CENTERED CARE

Part III NURSING CONSIDERATIONS FOR PEOPLE WITH DEMENTIA DURING SPECIFIC STAGES

Preface

If you are a nurse working in an adult health setting, you most likely care for patients whose mental status is altered. It is also likely that many of your patients who are older than 75 or 80 years have a diagnosis of dementia and others have manifestations of dementia but have not been "officially labeled" as such. In addition, if you work in an acute care setting, it is likely that many of your patients experience an altered mental status due to delirium. Despite the increasing awareness of delirium as a cause of altered mental status, many of these patients will not be diagnosed as such. In all these circumstances, one of your primary nursing responsibilities is to address the needs of patients whose mental status is compromised, whether it is due to dementia, delirium, or a combination of these conditions.

Fast Facts for Dementia Care has evolved out of more than four decades of my gerontological nursing experiences caring for people with dementia in a wide range of clinical settings, including acute care, long-term care, and home and community settings. Its intent is to help you incorporate a person-centered approach in your usual nursing care as you address the unique needs of people who have dementia. The basic premise is that although the short-term nature of the care setting focuses on nursing interventions for immediate medical problems, nurses have numerous opportunities to incorporate dementia-specific interventions in care plans. This approach does not require extra time; in many circumstances, it saves time because it prevents problems from occurring or addresses issues before they escalate. These person-centered interventions for dementia can have a significant positive effect on the care you provide. In addition, if you are familiar with the dementia-related issues and resources discussed in this book, you have numerous opportunities to suggest referrals for longer-term follow-up.

Chapters in Part I discuss types of dementia and other commonly occurring conditions that have similar manifestations; these chapters focus on nursing responsibilities for assessment and management of patients whose mental status is altered by underlying conditions such as dementia or delirium. Chapters in Part II describe how nurses can apply a person-centered approach to address dementia-related issues. Part III discusses nursing care issues at various stages of dementia, and Part IV provides information about addressing emotional and behavioral issues. Chapters in Part V describe considerations related to specific care settings and provide information about nursing strategies for daily care, safety, and pain management. Chapters in Part VI are a guide to broader aspects of care for people with dementia, including self-neglect and elder abuse and ethical and legal issues. The last chapter discusses nursing strategies to address the needs of caregivers of people with dementia. A major emphasis throughout the text is on relatively simple interventions that nurses can incorporate in their discharge plans to teach families and care partners about sources of information and support to address the needs of people with dementia.

Although some terminology in this book may seem cumbersome or unfamiliar, I have made every effort to use terms that are consistent with my focus on person-centered care. For example, I consistently use the phrase *person with dementia* to emphasize the personhood of the patient who has dementia as a chronic condition affecting his or her care. I also use the term *care partners* to emphasize that people with dementia are not passive recipients of care, particularly during mild and moderate stages. This phrase is appropriate because the care of people with dementia requires the *partnership* of many personal and professional support people working together to address this complex situation. The term *caregiver* is used in some chapters in reference to the needs of family members and support people who are most directly affected, particularly when the person has moderate or severe dementia.

Many years ago, one of my clients told me, "I try to learn from my dementia so I can help others." This client is one of the hundreds of individuals with dementia who have enhanced my professional nursing education and research as I have developed my expertise in dementia. As a geriatric care manager, I have often advocated for my clients when they receive care in hospitals, EDs, their homes, and long-term care settings. In all these settings, I have discussed their care with nurses who are experts in addressing medical issues but have little knowledge about addressing issues that arise out of their patients' dementia. In this book, I share the expertise I have developed so nurses in all settings can address the unique and challenging needs of their patients who are individuals with dementia. It is my hope that the information in this book will not only improve care for people with dementia but also improve professional life for nurses who care for them.

Carol A. Miller

Acknowledgments

First and foremost, I appreciate the many people with dementia and their families and care partners whom I have cared for and care about as a nurse. I value the challenges they have presented and the opportunities I have had for applying my expertise and learning from them. I am grateful for Pat Rehm's unending support and understanding as I have engaged in this writing venture, and I also appreciate my family cheerleaders who provide many expressions of encouragement. Finally, I extend my deepest appreciation to Elizabeth Nieginski and Rachel Landes and all those at Springer Publishing Company who guided this book from idea to reality.

1

Dementia: What It Is, What It Is Not, and What Nurses Can Do

1

Dementia Overview

INTRODUCTION

Minor changes in cognitive function are a normal part of healthy aging; however, any cognitive impairments that significantly interfere with usual daily functioning or quality of life are caused by underlying pathological conditions. Nurses who provide care for older adults in any setting need to be knowledgeable about cognitive changes to accurately assess and address functioning and quality of life. This chapter presents information about normal cognitive aging and dementia and provides the foundation for incorporating a person-centered approach when you care for older adults who are cognitively compromised.

In this chapter, you will learn:

1. Normal cognitive aging and mild cognitive impairment
2. Definition and types of dementia
3. Conditions that are closely associated with dementia
4. How dementia is diagnosed
5. Stages of dementia
6. Roles of nurses in identifying dementia

NORMAL COGNITIVE AGING AND MILD COGNITIVE IMPAIRMENT

Cognitive changes that are an inherent part of aging do not significantly affect functioning, personality, or behavior. Moreover, not all cognitive changes are negative. Cognitive changes that healthy older adults commonly experience by the time they are in their 70s or 80s include the following:

- Improved wisdom, creativity, common sense, coordination of facts and ideas, and breadth of knowledge
- Difficulty finding the right word quickly
- Slower processing of information
- Increased difficulty with abstraction, calculation, word fluency, verbal comprehension, spatial orientation, and inductive reasoning
- Decreased memory for details of events of the past but no change in short-term memory

Mild cognitive impairment (MCI) has been used since the mid-1990s to describe **a state of cognitive function that lies between normal aging changes and dementia**. Identification of MCI is determined by the presence of impairment of one or more of the listed cognitive domains: memory, attention, visuospatial abilities, and executive functioning without major declines in overall cognition or daily functioning. Initially, MCI was considered a precursor to Alzheimer's disease but is now considered a distinct syndrome with symptoms that can resolve, remain stable, or progress.

When older adults experience cognitive changes that affect daily functioning, encourage them to obtain an assessment by a geriatric practitioner who is knowledgeable about cognitive aging, MCI, and dementia. In addition, the following adaptations are suggested to improve communication during healthcare interactions with older adults who are experiencing MCI:

- Provide small amounts of information at one time.
- Allow enough time for information processing.
- Use simple written and visual materials.
- Reinforce information with repetition.
- Ask for feedback to ascertain the person's understanding.

Fast Facts

Nurses can differentiate between normal and pathological cognitive changes by assessing the degree to which the changes affect functioning.

⟳ **Clinical Snapshot**

Normal cognitive aging may cause older adults to have momentary difficulty remembering where they left their car, but older adults who have dementia may not remember that they drove a car.

DEFINITION AND TYPES OF DEMENTIA

In the words of a person with dementia:

> I noticed a difficulty in remembering names. . . . This is what I was most worried about . . . because it wasn't well. . . . It was my memory, which is the part of my body that I have been working the most with. (Larsson, Holmbom-Larsen, & Torisson, 2019, p. 5)

Dementia refers to a group of brain disorders characterized by a progressive decline in cognitive abilities and changes in personality and behavior. Dementia typically begins with a gradual onset of manifestations that are difficult to distinguish from MCI.

Short-term memory impairment is the most widely recognized manifestation of dementia, but many other signs and symptoms occur. For example, personality changes that commonly begin early and may progress include declines in self-discipline and competence, decreased energy and assertiveness, and increased vulnerability to stress (Islam et al., 2019). As dementia progresses, the manifestations gradually affect all aspects of functioning, and eventually the condition is considered terminal.

Fast Facts

Rather than being a single disease, dementia is an umbrella term that indicates the presence of a constellation of manifestations indicative of a progressive neurodegenerative brain disease.

Alzheimer's disease, first described in medical literature in 1907, is the most common and widely recognized type of dementia. Alzheimer's disease is characterized by hallmark pathological changes that affect specific regions of the brain.

Vascular dementia, which was identified in the 1970s, is caused by the death of nerve cells in regions of the brain usually nourished by the affected blood vessels. This type is associated with major strokes or cumulative effects of many minor strokes. When vascular dementia is caused by a major stroke, it has an acute onset, does not always progress, and often improves with therapies. This type, therefore, may not fit the characteristics of gradual, progressive, and irreversible.

In recent decades, the increasing availability of data based on longitudinal studies and newer brain imaging techniques has facilitated the identification of other types of dementia, such as Lewy body dementia and frontotemporal dementia. **Lewy body dementia** is part of a group of disorders, including Parkinson's disease, that are associated with the accumulation of abnormal proteins (i.e., Lewy bodies) in the brain. **Frontotemporal dementia** describes a spectrum of neurodegenerative disorders, such as Pick's disease, involving the frontal or temporal lobes, or both. Manifestations of frontotemporal dementia often begin before the person is 60 years old and may be misidentified as a psychiatric disease.

Table 1.1 outlines distinguishing features of these four most commonly diagnosed types.

Table 1.1

Distinguishing Features of Four Major Types of Dementia	
Type	**Distinguishing Features**
Alzheimer's disease	Slow onset with gradual progression over 5–10 or more years; loss of short-term memory is a prominent characteristic that begins early and progresses throughout the course; gradual effects on personality, behavior, and all aspects of functioning.
Vascular dementia	Gradual onset due to cumulative effects of small strokes or sudden onset if related to a major stroke; typically associated with cardiovascular risk factors such as strokes, atrial fibrillation, coronary artery disease, and high blood pressure; irregular course or possible improvement depending on causative factors and presence of other brain pathologies.
Lewy body dementia	Has many manifestations that overlap with those of Alzheimer's disease or Parkinson's disease; fluctuating levels of cognition and overall functioning; characterized by complex visual hallucinations, sleep disturbances, and spontaneous motor parkinsonism.

(*continued*)

Table 1.1

Distinguishing Features of Four Major Types of Dementia (*continued*)

Frontotemporal dementia	Gradual onset between fifth and seventh decade with personality and behavioral changes (e.g., apathy, impulsivity, emotional lability, poor social skills); diminished concentration, attention, reasoning, and judgment; loss of speech and language skills; falls, gait changes, movement disorders, and muscle rigidity.

In the words of a person with dementia

> Yes, it is called Lewy body dementia but I think that's so rotten. . . .
> If you tell colleagues then they will put a mark in your forehead,
> or joke or something funny. . . . You have to protect yourself . . . in
> your soul . . . against this dementia mark. (Larsson et al., 2019, p. 4)

CONDITIONS THAT ARE CLOSELY ASSOCIATED WITH DEMENTIA

Some neurological conditions progress to the point that dementia develops in most patients with these diseases. For example, **dementia eventually develops in most patients with Parkinson's disease**, and conversely, Parkinson's-like motor disability commonly develops in patients with Lewy body or Alzheimer's dementia.

Other conditions that often progress to dementia:

- AIDS
- Multiple sclerosis
- Huntington's disease
- Creutzfeldt–Jakob disease
- Normal pressure hydrocephalus (NPH)
- Acute or chronic head trauma

These conditions typically impair some aspect of physical functioning prior to affecting cognition. Conditions that cause dementia-like symptoms and usually resolve when the underlying cause is treated are discussed in Chapter 2, Conditions That Affect Cognitive Function.

HOW DEMENTIA IS DIAGNOSED

In the words of a person with dementia:

> At the start of the test, I thought: Well, this is really a piece of cake. The questions and sums were so silly, so obvious! But at a certain point (*starts crying*) I noticed that it was not clear to me at all. (Van Wijngaarden, Alma, & The, 2019, p. 8)

There is **no single test for dementia**, and even the most skilled geriatric practitioners find that **it is challenging to diagnose dementia in its earliest stages**. Even upon diagnosis, it is difficult to identify the specific type because of overlapping or similar features. Moreover, an individual may have pathological changes and manifestations of two or more types of dementia at the same time. For example, studies suggest that more than half of the people with Lewy body dementia also have pathological changes associated with Alzheimer's disease (Chin, Teodorczuk, & Watson, 2019).

In general clinical settings, the **diagnosis of dementia is both retrospective and "rule-out."** It is retrospective because, with the exception of stroke-associated dementia, manifestations develop over many years; it is a rule-out process because the workup is directed toward identifying any treatable condition that can cause similar manifestations. A major clinical implication of an accurate diagnosis of dementia is that all treatable causes are identified as early as possible so that they can be addressed. In research settings, such as university-affiliated medical centers, the use of specialized neuroimaging techniques and other diagnostic measurements is improving the diagnosis of dementia and differentiation among the types even in early stages (Mahalingam & Chen, 2019).

A comprehensive evaluation for dementia is warranted under the following combination of circumstances:

- The cognitive or behavioral symptoms interfere with the usual activities.
- The changes represent a decline from the person's usual level of functioning.
- The manifestations are not due to conditions such as stroke, delirium, head trauma, medical conditions, psychiatric disorders, or adverse medication effects.

Exhibit 1.1 identifies the components of a comprehensive evaluation procedure for dementia in clinical settings.

Exhibit 1.1

Components of Dementia Evaluation

Dementia evaluation

- Is multidisciplinary, involving a team of geriatric healthcare professionals
- Considers changes that occur over months or years
- Is an ongoing process with intermittent reevaluations
- Includes direct observation and evaluations by healthcare professionals
- Includes appropriate inputs and observations from reliable family, friends, caregivers, and acquaintances

Essential components

- Comprehensive history of changes in cognition, personality, and behavior
- Complete physical examination to identify underlying medical conditions
- Functional assessment
- CT scan and MRI
- Neuropsychological testing

Components of neuropsychological testing

- Personality or behavioral changes, such as apathy, impulsivity, mood fluctuations, or socially inappropriate actions
- Memory skills
- Ability to acquire and remember new information
- Reasoning, judgment, or handling of complex tasks
- Visuospatial abilities
- Language and communication skills
- Affective changes, such as depression

Additional diagnostic tests used in specialized settings or for clinical research

- Fluorodeoxyglucose (FDG) PET
- Amyloid PET scans
- Tau PET scans
- Cerebrospinal fluid analysis
- Genetic testing

Fast Facts

Dementia is a very complex diagnosis that requires comprehensive evaluations of all aspects of functioning and an overview of changes over time (Exhibit 1.1).

STAGES OF DEMENTIA

Although specific characteristics are associated with each type of dementia, many characteristics are common to all types of dementia. Common characteristics of mild, moderate, and advanced stages of dementia are as follows:

Mild Dementia

- Cognitive impairments that interfere with the performance of familiar tasks
- Impaired judgment, problem-solving, and decision-making skills
- Difficulty processing visual or spatial information
- Significant problems with speaking or writing
- Withdrawal from usual work or social activities
- Changes in mood or personality (e.g., increased anxiety, irritability, depression)

Moderate Dementia

- Continued decline in all aspects of cognition
- Increasing confusion
- Need for some assistance or direction with usual activities
- Disorientation to time or place
- Frequent or intermittent occurrence of neuropsychological manifestations (e.g., delusions, hallucinations, agitation, depression, apathy)

Advanced Dementia

- Major impairments in all aspects of cognition
- Inability to recognize familiar people or surroundings
- Need for assistance in all activities of daily living
- Disrupted sleep/wake cycle

- Significant personality changes and behavioral manifestations (e.g., agitation, repetitive behaviors, delusions, hallucinations)
- Diminished physical functioning, including incontinence and impaired mobility

Keep in mind that **dementia is a progressive condition** affected by numerous interacting conditions and circumstances, such as concomitant medical conditions, environmental and psychosocial influences, and caregiver factors. In addition, **dementia affects people in individualized** ways. People with dementia do not fit neatly into categories.

Stages of dementia describe the progression of the condition and its effects on the person's functioning and are not related in any way to the person's age. The typical age for onset of dementia is during the seventh decade or later, but dementia can occur in people in their 40s or 50s also. When dementia occurs before the age of 60, it is called early-onset disease.

Fast Facts

Dementia progresses through mild, moderate, and advanced stages, and each stage is characterized by progressive changes in cognition, behavior, and functioning. However, the progression is not necessarily linear, and the person with dementia may experience fluctuations between the stages.

ROLES OF NURSES IN IDENTIFYING DEMENTIA

Nurses are not responsible for diagnosing dementia, but they are responsible for assessing changes in mental status during the course of usual nursing care. They are also **responsible for suggesting referrals for further evaluation when mental status is compromised** in any way. Every clinical setting has mental status assessment forms that generally include criteria such as orientation, alertness, and contact with reality (e.g., hallucinations). In addition, some clinical settings use standardized mental status assessment forms, such as the mini–mental status examination or the Montreal Cognitive Assessment. No matter what assessment format is used, additional assessment skills are necessary because the assessment tools do not identify underlying conditions that affect mental status.

When caring for a person who has been diagnosed with dementia, **identify concomitant conditions that may be affecting behavior and mental status** rather than attributing the change to a manifestation of dementia. Be on the alert for treatable components whenever the person with dementia experiences a change in functioning. For example, an infection or electrolyte imbalance can affect overall functioning and mental status in older adults, and nurses are in a key position to assess for these conditions and take appropriate action rather than attributing the changes to dementia. Chapter 2, Conditions That Affect Cognitive Function, and Chapter 3, Nursing Assessment of and Interventions for Delirium, discuss many of the conditions that affect people with dementia or those that are mistakenly attributed to dementia.

Fast Facts

In addition to using standard mental status assessment forms, assess for conditions that affect cognitive function, especially those that can be addressed through nursing interventions.

⚙ Clinical Snapshot: Through the Stages of Dementia

Mild Dementia
During the past few years, Sophie D, a 73-year-old widow living alone, has become more and more forgetful about keeping appointments. In contrast to her previous meticulous mode of personal care, she no longer washes her hair and wears soiled and mismatched clothes. She has difficulty shopping for groceries and now walks to the nearby fast-food stores for most of her meals. The family has noticed that she no longer sends birthday cards to grandchildren as she has faithfully done for many years. She has little awareness of these changes and, in fact, is quite defensive when anyone questions her about memory problems.

Moderate Dementia

Sophie is now 76 years old and has recently moved to an assisted living facility because she did not take her medications for blood pressure and frequently fell and did not call for help when she could not get up. Staff members provide direction or assistance for all activities of daily living, including giving her medications, setting out her clothing every morning, and reminding her about using the toilet every few hours. She attends group activities a couple of times a day and especially enjoys the music events. She frequently asks about when her family will visit but does not

(continued)

(*continued*)

remember that she had visitors an hour ago. She spends much of her time looking for misplaced objects and sometimes takes things belonging to other residents and believes they are her own.

Advanced Dementia

Sophie is 81 years old and has moved to a memory-care nursing facility because she needs full assistance with all activities of daily living. She has lost weight and complains about the mechanical soft diet that is prescribed because of her difficulty with chewing and swallowing. When her family visits, she usually does not recognize them, but she says they are "very nice people." All cognitive skills are significantly impaired, and it is difficult to carry on a normal conversation. She has no memory for recent or remote events and often asks where her husband is, despite the fact that he has been dead for 16 years. She has difficulty walking and fallen a couple of times because she does not call for help when she needs to get out of bed.

References

Chin, K. S., Teodorczuk, A., & Watson, R. (2019). Dementia with Lewy bodies: Challenges in the diagnosis and management. *Australia and New Zealand Journal of Psychiatry, 53*(4), 291–303. doi:10.1177/0004867419835029

Islam, M., Mazumder, M., Schwabe-Warf, D., Stephan, Y., Sutin, A. R., & Terracciano, A. (2019). Personality changes with dementia from the informant perspective: New data and meta-analysis. *Journal of the American Medical Directors Association, 20*(2), 131–137. doi:10.1016/j.jamda.2018.11.004

Larsson, V., Holmbom-Larsen, A., Torisson, G., Strandberg, E. L., & Londos, E. (2019). Living with dementia with Lewy bodies: An interpretive phenomenological analysis. *BMJ Open, 9*(1), e024983. doi:10.1136/bmjopen-2018-024983

Mahalingam, S., & Chen, M. K. (2019). Neuroimaging in dementias. *Seminars in Neurology, 39*(2), 188–199. doi:10.1055/s-0039-1678580

Van Wijngaarden, E., Alma, M., & The, A-M. (2019). "The eyes of others" are what really matters: The experience of living with dementia from an insider perspective. *PLoS ONE, 14*(4), e0214724. doi:10.1371/journal.pone.0214724

RESOURCES

Alzheimer's Association

www.alz.org

- Alzheimer's disease, including local resources for professionals and caregivers

HelpGuide

www.helpguide.org

- Information about age-related memory loss, types of dementia, and other pertinent topics

Lewy Body Dementia Association

www.lbda.org

- Information and resources about Lewy body dementia for professionals and caregivers

National Institute on Aging

www.nia.nih.gov/health/alzheimers

- Research and information about Alzheimer's disease and other dementias

National Institutes of Neurological Disorders and Stroke

www.ninds.nih.gov/disorders

- Information about stroke and types of dementia

Veterans Administration

https://www.va.gov/GERIATRICS/Alzheimers_and_Dementia_Care.asp

- Information about dementia and resources for care5

2

Conditions That Affect Cognitive Function

INTRODUCTION

Older adults experience age-related changes or mild cognitive impairment (MCI), but these changes do not significantly affect usual daily functioning. This chapter reviews conditions that can cause significant changes in cognitive function and affect usual functioning, with particular attention to those that can be addressed to prevent or reverse cognitive impairment. The manifestations of these conditions are sometimes mistakenly attributed to either "normal aging" or dementia, with the consequence of having treatable conditions left unrecognized and untreated. Thus, nurses have important responsibilities to assess for conditions that affect cognitive function and facilitate referrals for further evaluation.

In this chapter, you will learn:

1. Conditions that affect cognitive function
2. Medical conditions that can cause mental changes
3. Medications that can cause mental changes
4. Depression and dementia

5. Roles of nurses in identifying conditions that affect cognitive function
6. Nursing strategies to address conditions that affect cognitive function

CONDITIONS THAT CAN AFFECT COGNITIVE FUNCTION

Older adults are likely to experience age-related conditions that affect cognitive function and interfere with daily functioning. For example, longitudinal studies indicate that older adults with hearing and visual impairments are at an increased risk for MCI and dementia (Brenowitz, Kaup, Lin, & Yaffe, 2019; Maharani et al., 2019). In recent years, there is increasing attention to age-related hearing loss as a potentially reversible cause of dementia (Curhan, Willett, Grodstein, & Curhan, 2019; Uchida et al., 2019). Attention is also being paid to ototoxic medications as a risk for developing hearing loss and cognitive impairment.

Medications Identified as Potentially Ototoxic

- Loop diuretics
- Nonsteroidal anti-inflammatory drugs
- Antibiotics
- Chemotherapeutic agents
- Quinine
- Acetaminophen (Joo et al., 2020)

Additional conditions that often negatively impact cognitive function include **physical discomfort** (e.g., pain), **adverse medication effects**, and **psychosocial issues** (e.g., depression, social isolation). Although these conditions can affect people of any age, older adults are more likely to experience these conditions and more vulnerable to negative consequences when the conditions occur. In addition, age-related changes in cognitive function can affect the ability of older adults to process information. In clinical settings, nurses have important roles in teaching older adults about interventions that address conditions affecting cognitive function, as described in Table 2.1.

Fast Facts

Nurses have many opportunities in clinical settings to directly address cognitive changes, and they can teach about interventions the older adult can use (see Table 2.1).

Table 2.1

Nursing Strategies to Support Good Cognitive Function in Clinical Settings

Condition	Nursing Strategies
Impaired vision	Use visual aids with large-type and good-contrast letters and pictures. Provide adequate nonglare lighting. Encourage eye examinations as appropriate. Ensure the glasses are accessible and clean if the person wears eyeglasses.
Impaired hearing	Position yourself face-to-face with the patient. Reduce background noise as much as possible. Pace your speech appropriately. Use amplifier device if needed. Articulate words, but do not exaggerate. Do not chew gum while talking. Make sure hearing aids are available and functional if the person uses a hearing aid. Encourage hearing evaluation as appropriate.
Physical discomfort	Ensure as much comfort as possible by addressing pain, thirst, hunger, discomfort, fatigue, and other conditions.
Medications	Assess and address medication effects that may interfere with cognitive function (e.g., the anticholinergic effects of many medications can compromise mental status).
Emotional stress	Be fully present to the patient. Use good listening skills. Encourage patients to express feelings. Teach simple breathing exercises for stress reduction. Encourage the presence of supportive friends/family.

MEDICAL CONDITIONS THAT CAN CAUSE MENTAL CHANGES

Certain medical conditions can affect many aspects of brain functioning. When the conditions progress without being identified or treated, they can cause dementia-like mental changes. Conditions that develop slowly and have subtle manifestations include:

- Hypothyroidism
- Hyperthyroidism
- Anemia
- Vitamin B_{12} deficiency
- Infections (e.g., urinary tract infections)
- Repeated transient ischemic attacks (small vessel cerebrovascular disease)

Delirium is a commonly occurring medical condition characterized by significant mental status changes, and this topic is addressed in detail in Chapter 3, Nursing Assessment of and Interventions for Delirium.

Fast Facts

Poorly controlled chronic conditions can cause or contribute to altered mental status and may look like dementia.

⊙ Clinical Snapshot

Mrs. G is being evaluated for memory problems, which have worsened during the past 6 months. Her nutrition is poor, and she does not take her medications consistently. She had been taking levothyroxine (Synthroid) for many years, but you question whether she has been taking it, and you ask when was the last time she had her hypothyroidism evaluated.

MEDICATIONS THAT CAN CAUSE MENTAL CHANGES

Medications are a common cause of mental changes in older adults. People with dementia have the double risk of being more susceptible to adverse medication effects and having these effects inaccurately attributed to underlying dementia. Cumulative effects of **anticholinergic medications are one of the most common causes of serious mental changes** in all older adults, with increased risk among those with dementia. Drug interactions can potentiate the risk for mental changes, particularly when two or more drugs with anticholinergic action are taken. Alcohol abuse is also a common cause of mental changes that is often subtle or overlooked in older adults and people

Table 2.2

Adverse Medication Effects That Can Cause Mental Changes	
Type of Medication	**Example of Adverse Effect**
Anticholinergics	Neurological adverse effects, including cognitive impairment, slowed responses, and confusion
Diuretics, antidepressants	Hyponatremia
Diabetic medications	Hypoglycemia
Corticosteroids	Hyperglycemia, hormonal disturbances
Antipsychotics	Neurological adverse effects

with dementia. Table 2.2 lists other adverse medication effects that can cause mental changes, with examples of types of medications.

Fast Facts

Cumulative effects of medications, especially those with anticholinergic properties, can cause gradual mental changes that are inaccurately attributed to dementia.

Clinical Snapshot

After Mrs. P, who had taken hydrochlorothiazide (Diuril) for many years, began taking citalopram (Celexa) for depression, she became increasingly confused. Her serum sodium level was 127 mEq/L, which was attributed to two medications that can cause hyponatremia. Her mental status returned to normal after the medications were changed.

DEPRESSION AND DEMENTIA

Depression is increasingly being addressed as a commonly occurring condition that is a serious and treatable cause of cognitive changes. People with dementia have a **higher incidence of depression** but are more likely to have it overlooked as a separate and treatable condition. Depression is not a normal part of aging, but it occurs commonly in older adults due to the increased number of risk factors.

Depression Risk Factors

- Cumulative or chronic stressors (e.g., losses, caregiver demands)
- Loss of social support
- Medical conditions, including stroke, dementia, cancer, myocardial infarction, and Parkinson's disease
- Functional limitations (especially recent onset)
- New medical diagnosis
- Chronic pain
- Alcohol or substance abuse

Consequences of depression include an increased risk for developing dementia, significantly diminished quality of life, and increased risk for committing suicide.

Dementia complicates the diagnosis of depression because the two conditions have overlapping manifestations, such as:

- Impaired memory
- Poor concentration
- Difficulty making decisions
- Withdrawal from social activity
- Apathy (i.e., lack of motivation and initiation)
- Irritability
- Personality changes

Table 2.3

Distinguishing Features of Dementia and Depression		
Characteristic	**Dementia**	**Depression**
Onset	Gradual, recognized by hindsight	Rapid, often associated with a triggering event
Awareness	Unaware or minimizes the symptoms	Exaggerated perception of cognitive deficits
Memory and attention	Impaired memory and attention, but strong attempts to perform well	Cognitive deficits due to lack of motivation and inability to concentrate
Emotions	Affect changes easily in response to suggestions	Consistent feelings of sadness; tearfulness is common
Response to questions	Inaccurate but attempts to cover up deficits	Minimal response with little or no effort put forth
Decision-making	Impaired due to difficulty processing information	Impaired due to lack of motivation
Personal appearance	Inappropriate dress due to impaired perceptions and thought processes	Little or no concern about appearance because of lack of motivation
Physical complaints	Inconsistent and vague complaints (e.g., tired, weak)	Sleep disturbances, gastrointestinal complaints, decreased energy
Social interaction	Enjoys social interaction and activities if they are not too challenging	Withdrawal from usual activities due to lack of enjoyment
Contact with reality	Misinterpretation of reality; if present, delusions are aimed at explaining deficits	Exaggerated sense of gloom and doom; auditory hallucinations or self-derogatory delusions

Despite the similarities, nurses can differentiate between these two conditions by considering the distinguishing characteristics of dementia and depression described in Table 2.3.

Fast Facts

Nurses can differentiate between dementia and depression by assessing a person's response to questions.

Clinical Snapshot

When you ask Mr. D (who has mild dementia) if he has noticed any changes in his memory, he replies, "I can tell you everything you'd ever want to know about the invasion of Normandy in World War II." When you ask Mrs. G (who is depressed) if she has noticed any changes in her memory, she replies, "I've been forgetting my appointments for lunch with friends, but that's okay because I've been staying in bed till afternoon."

ROLES OF NURSES IN IDENTIFYING CONDITIONS THAT AFFECT COGNITIVE FUNCTION

Take a detective-like approach to identifying conditions that can be mistakenly attributed to dementia. Obtain information about the person's usual mental status so that changes can be identified for further evaluation and possible interventions. Whenever a change in mental status is noted, obtain the following information:

- Diagnostic measures that have been taken to identify medical conditions
- Management of chronic conditions, such as diabetes, thyroid disorders, or congestive heart failure
- Prescription and nonprescription medications being taken
- Recent changes in medications (new prescriptions and discontinuation of medications)
- Possible drug interactions, particularly with recently prescribed medications
- Use of alcohol or recreational substances (or withdrawal from these)

In addition to identifying physiological conditions that affect mental status, **assess for depression**. The American Geriatrics Society recommends periodic depression screening for all people beginning at age 60 and every 6 months for older persons with dementia. Many healthcare settings have easy-to-use depression screening tools, such as the Geriatric Depression Scale, which can be administered in 5 to 7 minutes. The resources section at the end of this chapter provides information about this and other screening tools. The U.S. Preventive Services Task Force (2009) recommends the following two questions to identify depression:

- During the past 2 weeks (or month), have you felt down, depressed, or hopeless?
- During the past 2 weeks (or month), have you felt little interest or pleasure in doing things?

An affirmative response to either of these questions calls for further assessment with a formal depression scale.

NURSING STRATEGIES TO ADDRESS CONDITIONS THAT AFFECT COGNITIVE FUNCTION

Nurses in short-term settings have limited opportunity to directly address conditions that look like dementia. However, they can take the following actions:

- Facilitate referrals for further evaluation immediately or after discharge.
- Raise questions about adverse medication effects or drug interactions that can cause or contribute to mental changes.
- Refer for social work assistance with plans for follow-up.
- If specialized geriatric services are available within the institution (as discussed in Chapter 9, Caring for the Person With Advanced Dementia), follow the procedure for a referral.
- If there are indicators that the person is depressed, teach about the importance of having depression evaluated and refer to social worker for follow-up.
- Teach persons with dementia and their care partners about reversible and treatable conditions that mimic dementia.

Fast Facts

Be aware of opportunities to detect depression in people with dementia so you can initiate interventions.

⟳ Clinical Snapshot

Mr. T, who has been admitted for exacerbation of congestive heart failure, expresses pervasive feelings of sadness and hopelessness. In addition, his wife reports that he has become more confused recently, even though he is on medications for dementia. After 3 days, his primary care practitioner says he is ready for discharge because his cardiac status is stable. You talk with Mr. and Mrs. T about depression and other conditions that can mimic dementia, and you provide contact information for further evaluation with the comprehensive geriatric assessment program.

References

Brenowitz, W. D., Kaup, A. R., Lin, F. R., & Yaffe, K. (2019). Multiple sensory impairment is associated with increased risk of dementia among black and white older adults. *Journals of Gerontology Series A: Biological Sciences and Medical Sciences, 74*(6), 890–896. doi:10.1093/gerona/gly/264

Curhan, S. G., Willett, W. C., Grodstein, F., & Curhan, G. C. (2019). Longitudinal study of hearing loss and subjective cognitive function decline in men. *Alzheimers Dementia, 15*(4), 525–533. doi:10.1016/j.jalz.2018.11.004

Joo, Y., Cruickshanks, K. J., Klein, B. E. K., Klein, R., Hong, O., & Wallhagen, M. I. (2020). The contribution of ototoxic medications to hearing loss among older adults. *Journals of Gerontology Series A: Biological Sciences and Medical Sciences, 75*(3), 561–566. doi:10.1093/gerona/glz166

Maharani, A., Dawes, P., Nazroo, J., Tampubolon, G., & Pendleton, N.; Sense-Cog WP1 Group. (2019). Associations between self-reported sensory impairment and risk of cognitive decline and impairment in the Health and Retirement Study (HRS) cohort. *Journals of Gerontology Series B: Psychological Sciences and Social Sciences.* doi:10.1093/geronb/gbzo43

Uchida, Y., Saguira, S., Nichita, Y., Saji, N., Sone, M., & Ueda, H. (2019). Age-related hearing loss and cognitive decline—The potential mechanisms linking the two. *Auris Nsaus Larynx, 46*(1), 1–9. doi:10.1016/j.anl.2018.08.010

U.S. Preventive Services Task Force. (2009). Screening for depression in adults: U.S. Preventive Services Task Force recommendation statement. *Annals of Internal Medicine, 151*(11), 784–792. doi:10.7326/0003-4819-151-11-200912010-00006

RESOURCES

Stanford University

www.stanford.edu/~yesavage/GDS.html

- Geriatric Depression Scale

Hartford Institute for Geriatric Nursing

https://consultgerirn.org

- The Geriatric Depression Scale, *Try This*, Issue 4, and video illustrating application of the assessment tool

Mayo Clinic

https://www.mayoclinic.org/diseases-conditions/dementia/symptoms-causes/syc-20352013

- Causes of dementia that can be reversed

3

Nursing Assessment of and Interventions for Delirium

INTRODUCTION

Delirium is increasingly being addressed in healthcare settings as a commonly occurring condition that is serious, preventable, treatable, and often unrecognized. In addition, it can have serious consequences—including death—when it is not recognized and addressed. Older adults with dementia have the double disadvantage of having a higher incidence of delirium and having it overlooked as a separate and treatable condition.

In this chapter, you will learn:

1. Definition and types of delirium
2. Predisposing and precipitating conditions associated with delirium
3. Medications as a cause of delirium
4. Consequences associated with delirium
5. Delirium superimposed on dementia
6. Roles of nurses in identifying conditions associated with delirium
7. Roles of nurses in addressing the needs of patients with delirium

DEFINITION AND TYPES OF DELIRIUM

Delirium is a medical syndrome characterized by:

- Abrupt change in mental status
- Abnormal level of consciousness
- Fluctuations in mental status
- Disturbances in thought, memory, attention, behavior, perception, and orientation
- Evidence of concomitant physiologic condition

Recent studies indicate that motor dysfunction (e.g., impaired balance and mobility) is another characteristic of delirium in people who also have dementia (Gual et al., 2019). Types of delirium are hypoactive (lethargic, stuporous), hyperactive (agitated, restless), and mixed (fluctuating between hypoactive and hyperactive). Hypoactive type is likely to be unrecognized because manifestations are not consistent with the usual perception of delirium as a hyperactive state.

PREDISPOSING AND PRECIPITATING CONDITIONS ASSOCIATED WITH DELIRIUM

Delirium results from an interaction between predisposing factors (i.e., characteristics that increase the person's vulnerability) and precipitating factors (i.e., conditions that are associated with the immediate threat). **Dementia is a major predisposing factor** that accounts for 65% of the incidence of delirium in hospital settings (Jackson et al., 2017). Studies indicate that people with more predisposing conditions are likely to develop delirium when only one or two precipitating factors occur (Oh & Park, 2019).

It is necessary to frequently assess for delirium in patients with dementia combined with additional risk factors. Exhibit 3.1 lists predisposing and precipitating conditions for the onset of delirium along with exacerbating conditions that worsen the delirium. Although predisposing conditions cannot be reversed, healthcare professionals need to identify these as risks for delirium, particularly in patients who have dementia. Precipitating conditions can be addressed through multidisciplinary interventions, as discussed in the section "Roles of Nurses in Identifying Conditions Associated With Delirium."

Exhibit 3.1

Conditions Associated With Increased Risk for Delirium

Predisposing factors (generally chronic conditions)

- Dementia
- History of delirium
- Age 70 or older
- Increased number of medical conditions
- Polypharmacy, especially drugs with anticholinergic effects
- Functional impairment
- Vision or hearing impairment
- Depression
- Malnutrition, vitamin deficiency

Precipitating factors (generally acute conditions)

- Pain
- Infections
- Anesthesia
- Surgery (especially cardiac or orthopedic)
- Medications, especially those with anticholinergic effects
- Falls
- Fluid or electrolyte imbalances (e.g., hyponatremia, hypokalemia, elevated glucose)
- Physiologic disturbances (e.g., hypoxia, dehydration)

Exacerbating conditions (those that occur after onset of delirium and worsen the manifestations)

- Environmental conditions, especially in acute-care settings (e.g., overstimulation, noise, lights)
- Lack of personal aids for sensory impairment (e.g., eyeglasses and hearing aids)
- Sleep deprivation
- Anxiety
- Inactivity, bedrest

Fast Facts

Whenever changes in mental status are observed in people with dementia, check for signs of delirium.

MEDICATIONS AS A CAUSE OF DELIRIUM

Medications are strongly associated with incidence of delirium, as both predisposing and precipitating factors (see Table 3.1). For example, **medications with strong anticholinergic effects** can predispose to delirium through neurologic adverse effects and also be a precipitating condition when an additional anticholinergic medication is prescribed. In addition to these direct effects, medication can predispose to or precipitate delirium by causing physiologic imbalances, such as dehydration or hyponatremia.

Although most nurses do not prescribe medications, **all nurses are responsible for assessing for altered mental status** as an adverse effect. Nurses can apply the following guidelines to assess medications as a condition that contributes to delirium:

Table 3.1

Medications That Can Cause Delirium	
Type	**Example**
Preanesthesia drugs	Atropine (Atropen), scopolamine (Hyoscine)
Bladder antispasmodics	Oxybutynin (Ditropan)
Antihistamines	Chlorpheniramine (Chlor-Trimeton), diphenhydramine (Benadryl)
Antianxiety agents	Benzodiazepines (e.g., Valium, Xanax)
Antipsychotics	Chlorpromazine (Thorazine), fluphenazine (Prolixin)
Antidepressants	Amitriptyline (Elavil), imipramine (Tofranil)
Movement disorders	Benztropine (Cogentin), trihexphenidyl (Artane)
Cardiovascular drugs	Disopyramide (Norpace), digitalis (Digoxin), propranolol (Inderal)
Motion sickness, nausea	Meclizine (Antivert), promethazine (Phenergan)
Muscle spasm	Methocarbamol (Robaxin)
Analgesics, especially narcotics	Meperidine (Demerol)
Gastrointestinal agents	Dicyclomine (Bentyl), cimetidine (Tagamet)

- Be on the alert for drug interactions and recognize that any physiologic substance—including food, fluids, herbs, vitamins, alcohol, nicotine, and nonprescription medications—can alter medication effects.
- Check for recent changes in medication regimen, but recognize that some drugs that have been taken for a long time can cause delirium at any time, especially in conjunction with other physiologic alterations.
- Recognize that older adults are more susceptible to medication-induced delirium because of age-related changes in the brain.
- Recognize that acute and chronic medical conditions are associated with increased risk for developing delirium.
- Recognize that a change in mental status can be caused by withdrawal from prescribed medications, illegal drugs, or alcohol.
- Obtain serum levels of medications that should be monitored.
- Avoid using medications for addressing behavioral issues that can be resolved with nonpharmacological interventions.

CONSEQUENCES ASSOCIATED WITH DELIRIUM

Delirium is associated with serious consequences for the patient, the family caregivers, and the healthcare setting including the following:

- Longer hospital stays
- Increased death rate
- Increased dependency and functional impairment
- Increased risk of long-term cognitive impairment
- Exacerbation of dementia
- Acceleration of cognitive decline
- Higher use of physical restraints
- Higher rates of permanent residency in long-term care facilities

Fast Facts

People with dementia have a triple disadvantage: They are more likely to develop delirium; they are less likely to have it diagnosed in a timely manner, and they are more likely to experience serious consequences.

DELIRIUM SUPERIMPOSED ON DEMENTIA

Because **impaired cognitive function is an inherent characteristic of both dementia and delirium,** it is difficult to distinguish between these two conditions. Dementia predisposes older adults to delirium and increases the risk that delirium will not be recognized and treated. Because dementia inherently involves altered cognitive function and an unpredictable course, **signs of delirium may be falsely attributed to the underlying dementia**. Table 3.2 summarizes distinguishing features of dementia and delirium.

Know the person's usual level of cognitive function and observe for even subtle changes associated with treatable conditions. Ask family members and care partners about the person's usual level of functioning and document this information to identify changes.

The Confusion Assessment Method (Inouye et al., 1990) is an easy-to-use standardized tool widely used by nurses in institutional settings to identify delirium (Exhibit 3.2). Additional related resources, including models for people with dementia and in intensive care units, are listed in the Resources section.

Table 3.2

Distinguishing Features of Dementia and Delirium		
Characteristic	**Dementia**	**Delirium**
Onset	Gradual	Sudden
Development	Slowly progressive over years	Rapid changes over hours
Attention	Usually can focus on task	Noticeably impaired, easily distracted
Consciousness	Alert and stable	Impaired and fluctuating
Speech	Confused but consistent	Incoherent
Course	Progressive, irreversible	Reversible if all causes are treated

Exhibit 3.2

Confusion Assessment Method (CAM) for Diagnosing Delirium

CONFUSION ASSESSMENT METHOD (CAM)

Features 1 and 2 plus 3 OR 4 indicates delirium

1. ACUTE ONSET AND
   FLUCTUATING COURSE

2. INATTENTION

AND

Change from baseline
Fluctuating behaviors

Difficulty focusing
Easily distracted

AND   3. DISORGANIZED THINKING
Rambling or irrelevant conversation
Unclear or illogical flow
Unpredictable change of topics

OR

4. ALTERED LEVEL OF CONSCIOUSNESS
Hyperalert, lethargic, stupor, or coma

ROLES OF NURSES IN IDENTIFYING CONDITIONS ASSOCIATED WITH DELIRIUM

The onset or progression of physiological disorders can precipitate delirium, and this may be more difficult to detect in people with dementia who cannot communicate accurately about their symptoms. Thus, **obtain objective information as well as reported information** from the person with dementia and that person's care partners. Figure 3.1 illustrates a flowchart for nursing assessment and interventions related to delirium.

Infections

Infections—including pneumonia, dental abscesses, and urinary tract infections—are the **most common causes of delirium.** Identification of infection in people with dementia is not straightforward for the following reasons: (a) they may not be able to accurately report their symptoms; (b) if their baseline temperature is low, which is common among older adults, their temperature may register as normal but be elevated above their usual; and (c) older adults may have a delayed or absent temperature elevation when they have an infection.

Nursing actions to detect infections include the following:

- Assess for pain, discomfort, and other physical changes.
- Check temperature for an increase above the baseline.
- Check urine specimen for indicators of urinary tract infection.
- Note any changes in urinary elimination (e.g., incontinence, frequency, or urgency).
- Assess skin, joints, and oral cavity for inflammation or recent onset of abnormalities.
- Assess respirations and lung sounds.
- Observe for changes in mobility or any aspect of functioning.
- Obtain orders for blood tests, sputum cultures, and chest x-rays as appropriate.

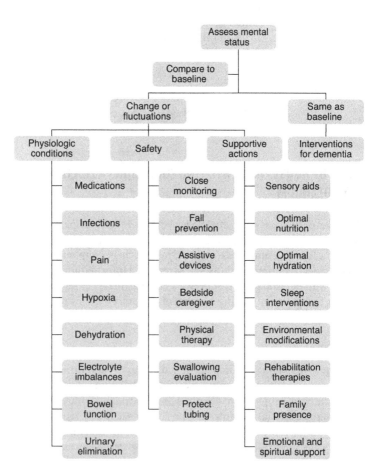

Figure 3.1 Flowchart for delirium.

Fast Facts

What is the rationale for obtaining a urinalysis when a change in a patient's behavior is noted? Rationale: A urinary tract infection is a common cause of delirium in older adults.

Physiologic Alterations

Other physiologic alterations that cause delirium include hypoxia, dehydration, malnutrition, fecal impactions, hypo- or hyperglycemia, and electrolyte imbalances. The following nursing actions assess for physiologic alterations:

- Assess all vital signs.
- Check pulse oximetry.
- Check blood glucose with glucometer.
- Review lab work, including electrolytes and blood counts, and obtain orders for appropriate tests.
- Monitor intake and output.
- Assess nutritional status.
- Check bowel sounds.
- Obtain information about recent bowel movements.
- Perform digital rectal examination for fecal impaction.
- Assess skin, oral mucous membrane, and urine specific gravity for indications of dehydration.

Fast Facts

Take a detective-like approach to identify conditions that may be causing delirium.

☼ Clinical Snapshot

Mr. M lives with his wife, who reported that the police brought him home after he had gone outside during the night in his pajamas. When the visiting nurse assessed him, she could find no signs of infection, but Mrs. M reported that a crown had fallen off one of her husband's teeth. Based on the nurse's advice, Mrs. M took her husband to his dentist, who found that he had an abscessed tooth. After the dental issue resolved, Mr. M had no further episodes of leaving the house at night.

Fast Facts

Combined effects of several anticholinergic medications can cause delirium.

◉ Clinical Snapshot

Mrs. N was brought to the ED for evaluation of recent-onset confusion. She has been taking oxybutynin (Ditropan) for overactive bladder and recently started taking Tylenol PM (acetaminophen and diphenhydramine/Benadryl) at bedtime and again during the night for difficulty sleeping due to arthritis pain. The geriatrician discontinued the oxybutynin and prescribed darifenacin (Enablex) and instructed Mrs. N to take plain acetaminophen at bedtime. Mrs. N's mental status returned to normal within a couple of days.

ROLES OF NURSES IN ADDRESSING NEEDS OF PATIENTS WITH DELIRIUM

Safety

Delirium in people with dementia is associated with significant personal safety risks, such as falls and aspiration pneumonia. These **risks are magnified if the person is unable to recognize the need for help or unable to use call lights or other devices** to obtain help in a timely manner. Delirium also increases the risk for the patient removing tubes connected with medically important, even life-sustaining, devices. The following nursing actions promote safety for people with dementia:

- Position patient close to the nursing station and monitor frequently.
- Arrange for bedside caregiver or family attendant to observe behaviors, prevent injuries, protect medical tubing, and provide cognitive and emotional support (e.g., orientation, reassurance, information).
- Obtain physical therapy evaluation and follow recommendations related to mobility assistance and use of assistive devices.
- Avoid the use of physical restraints and follow institutional policies for fall prevention.
- Use soft items or mittens to prevent the patient from pulling tubes out.

- Obtain swallowing evaluation and follow speech therapist's guidelines for safe eating and drinking techniques (e.g., thickened liquids, use of straws).

Fast Facts

Interventions for safety must be individualized and address the changes associated with both dementia and delirium.

✪ Clinical Snapshot

Mr. F uses a walker for safe mobility, but when he is in the hospital with delirium, he forgets to call for help and will get out of bed if he sees his walker. The nursing staff keep the walker out of sight because he does remember to call for help to find his walker.

Comfort and Physical Needs

Be proactive in addressing physical needs because **dementia and delirium compromise one's ability to ask for assistance**. Provide supportive interventions to address the emotional and spiritual needs of persons with dementia and their care partners. Nursing actions to address these needs include the following:

- Assess and address pain (see Chapter 15, Nursing Assessment and Management of Pain in People With Dementia).
- Obtain dietary consultations to address nutritional and hydration issues.
- Provide appropriate amounts of preferred foods and beverages and ensure that these are readily accessible.
- Provide good oral and skin care.
- Ensure access to sensory aids (e.g., clean eyeglasses, hearing devices).
- Limit noise as much as possible, but provide soothing music.
- Provide orientation reminders (clocks, calendars, up-to-date information on dry-erase boards).
- Obtain physical therapy for safe mobility and exercise program.
- Obtain occupational therapy for safety and independence in activities of daily living.
- Promote optimal urinary elimination (frequent assistance, timely response to requests for help, avoid the use of indwelling catheters).
- Promote optimal bowel elimination (measures to prevent or address constipation or diarrhea).

- Promote sleep (comfort measures, avoid sedatives/hypnotics).
- Obtain dental consultation to address issues with teeth, dentures, or oral cavity.
- Provide emotional support (listening, presence, encourage expression of feelings).
- Encourage presence of supportive care partners.
- Address spiritual needs.

References

Gual, N., Richardson, S., J., Davis, D. H. J., Bellelli, G., Hasemann, W., Meagher, D., & Morandi, A. (2019). Impairments in balance and mobility identify delirium in patients with comorbid dementia. *International Psychogeriatrics, 31*(5), 749–753. doi:10.1017/S104610218001345

Inouye, S., van Dyck, C., Alessi, C. A., Balkin, S., Siegal, A., & Horowitz, R. (1990). Clarifying confusion: The confusion assessment method. *Annals of Internal Medicine, 113*(12), 941–948. doi:10.7326/0003-4819-113-12-941

Jackson, T. A., Gladman, J. R., Harwood, R. H., MacLullich, A. M. J., Sampson, E. L., Sheehan, B., & Davis, D. H. J. (2017). Challenges and opportunities in understanding dementia and delirium in the acute hospital. *PLoS Medical, 14*(3), e1002247. doi:10.1371/journal.pmed.1002247

Oh, S-T., & Park, J. Y. (2019). Postoperative delirium. *Korean Journal of Anesthesiology, 72(1),* 4–12. doi:10.4097/kja.d.18.00073.1

RESOURCES

Hartford Institute for Geriatric Nursing

https://consultgerirn.org

- The Confusion Assessment Method (CAM), *Try This,* Issue 13, and video illustrating application of the assessment tool
- The Confusion Assessment Method for the ICU (CAM-ICU), *Try This,* Issue 25
- Assessing and Managing Delirium in Older Adults with Dementia, *Try This,* Issue D8
- Working with Families of Hospitalized Older Adults with Dementia, *Try This,* Issue D10

Critical Illness, Brain Dysfunction and Survivorship Center

https://www.icudelirium.org

- Information for professionals and families about delirium in the intensive care unit

4

Medical Management of Dementia

INTRODUCTION

For the past several decades, the medical management of dementia has been based on the use of two types of prescription drugs. Nurses often address questions about the use of these medications. They also address questions about the many nonprescription agents that are promoted for improving cognition not only for people with dementia but also for all adults for preventing dementia or improving cognitive function. This chapter provides an overview of current research and guidelines related to the medical management of dementia. The use of medications for dementia is one tiny aspect of the overall plan for managing dementia. Chapters in Part III, Nursing Considerations for People With Dementia During Specific Stages, and Part IV, Nursing Strategies to Address Emotional Needs and Behavioral Issues, provide detailed information about broader management issues related to dementia-related behaviors and quality of life, which are often the primary concerns when caring for people with dementia.

In this chapter, you will learn:

1. Medications approved for treatment of dementia
2. Nursing considerations about medications for dementia
3. Considerations for non-Alzheimer's dementia

4. Nonprescription agents
5. Medications for dementia-related symptoms
6. Nonpharmacologic interventions

MEDICATIONS APPROVED FOR TREATMENT OF DEMENTIA

Since the 1990s, three cholinesterase inhibitors and one N-methyl-D-aspartate (NMDA) antagonist have been widely prescribed for delaying or stabilizing the progression of some of the manifestations of dementia. Recent reviews of studies indicate that these drugs are associated with modest improvement in cognitive, functional, and behavioral manifestations of Alzheimer's disease, particularly during mild-to-moderate stages (Li, Zhang, Zhang, & Zhao, 2019). Reviews of recent studies also indicate that these drugs have similar effectiveness for vascular and Lewy body dementias (Jin & Liu, 2019; Meng, Wang, Song, & Wang, 2019). These drugs are not effective for frontotemporal dementia (Logroscino et al., 2019; Young, Lavakumar, Tampi, Balachandran, & Tampi, 2018). Although no new medication has been developed since 2003, newer dosing options are available for several of these medications. Table 4.1 summarizes actions, doses, and common side effects of medications for dementia.

Cholinesterase Inhibitors: Donepezil (Aricept), rivastigmine (Exelon), and galantamine (Razadyne, formerly called Reminyl). These medications:

- Increase levels of acetylcholine, a neurotransmitter that affects memory and cognition
- Are standard treatment to delay progression of symptoms of mild-to-moderate dementia; donepezil approved for all stages of dementia
- Are similar in therapeutic effectiveness (i.e., modest improvement or delay in progression of symptoms)
- Have similar side effects: nausea, diarrhea, vomiting, anorexia, weight loss
- Have less common side effects such as vivid dreams or nightmares, which can be addressed by reducing the dose or avoiding bedtime administration
- May differ in individual response to therapeutic and adverse effects
- Are started at a low dose and increased incrementally to prevent adverse effects and to reach optimal therapeutic levels
- Are less effective when anticholinergic medications are taken

Table 4.1

Medications Approved for Dementia			
Medication	**Action**	**Dose**	**Common Side Effects**
Donepezil (Aricept)	Prevents breakdown of acetylcholine in the brain	Begin with 5 mg once daily at bedtime; after 4–6 weeks, increase to 10 mg at bedtime as tolerated; after 3 months or more, increase to 23 mg for moderate-to-severe dementia	Nausea, vomiting, diarrhea, insomnia, loss of appetite
Rivastigmine (Exelon)	Prevents breakdown of acetylcholine and butyrylcholine in the brain	*Oral* (with full meal): Begin with 1.5 mg twice daily; at 2–4 week intervals, increase to 3 mg, 4.5 mg, and 6 mg twice daily as tolerated *Transdermal* (rotate sites): Begin with 4.6 mg daily; after 4–6 weeks, increase to 9.5 mg, then increase to 13.3 mg after 4–6 weeks	Nausea, vomiting, anorexia, diarrhea, weight loss, muscle weakness
Galantamine (Razadyne)	Prevents breakdown of acetylcholine and stimulates nicotinic receptors to release acetylcholine in the brain	Begin with 4 mg twice daily with food; at 4–6 week intervals, increase to 8 mg and 12 mg twice daily as tolerated; *extended release* form can be taken once daily	Nausea, vomiting, anorexia, weight loss
Memantine (Namenda)	Regulates glutamate activation and blocks toxic effects of excess glutamate	Begin with 5 mg once daily; at 1–2 week intervals, increase to 5 mg and 10 mg daily, then 10 mg twice daily as tolerated Extended release form begins at 7 mg once daily, with gradual increases to 28 mg per day	Dizziness, headache, constipation, hypertension

N-methyl-D-aspartate antagonist: memantine (Namenda). This medication:

- Regulates the level of the neurotransmitter glutamate in the brain, which is altered in dementia
- Is commonly used for moderate-to-severe dementia
- Has the therapeutic effect of a modest improvement or delay in progression of symptoms for about 6 months
- Should be used cautiously in people with severe renal disease, or in combination with amantadine (Symmetrel) or dextromethorphan (Delsym)

◑ Clinical Snapshot

Mrs. H began taking donepezil when she was first diagnosed with dementia, but she experienced gastrointestinal effects and lost weight. The medication was discontinued, and after 2 weeks, she began using the rivastigmine patch, which she tolerated well. Two years later, memantine was added to her regimen.

NURSING CONSIDERATIONS ABOUT MEDICATIONS FOR DEMENTIA

Nurses have many opportunities to teach about medications for dementia, particularly for people with mild dementia and for care partners of people with all stages of dementia. Some points to emphasize are:

- Many studies indicate that cholinesterase inhibitors have modest effects in delaying the progression of dementia.
- Medications are most effective when started early in the course of the condition.
- People with manifestations of dementia should be evaluated for appropriate medication management by a geriatrician or at a geriatric assessment program.
- As dementia progresses, medications should be reevaluated.
- Memantine is the only medication approved as an "add-on" to cholinesterase inhibitors for moderate-to-severe stages.

- Medications for dementia are started at low doses and increased gradually because adverse effects tend to diminish and the dose can be increased to therapeutic levels.
- It is important to follow the recommended titration doses and allow adequate time between dose adjustments.
- If compliance is difficult to achieve with pills, consider using transdermal patches (rivastigmine), once-daily dosing (donepezil, galantamine-ER), disintegrating sublingual tablets (donepezil), or a flavored liquid form (rivastigmine, memantine).
- If medications are not taken for several days, retitration may be necessary.
- Because these medications slow the progression of symptoms but do not otherwise alter the course of dementia, it is difficult to evaluate their effectiveness.

⟳ Clinical Snapshot

Mrs. W is being admitted for rehabilitation following knee replacement surgery. She states, "I've been having memory problems for about a year and my doctor told me I should take a medication for Alzheimer's, but I haven't started because my friend took something for that and then she lost a lot of weight." You respond, "There are several medications that are helpful for Alzheimer's, and they don't all have the same side effects. In fact, one of the medications can be used as a patch so it wouldn't affect your appetite or stomach. I suggest that you talk again with your doctor about trying one of these medications because they can slow the progression of your memory problem."

CONSIDERATIONS FOR NON-ALZHEIMER'S DEMENTIA

More information is available for Alzheimer's disease than for other types of dementia, but information related to specific types of dementia is increasing rapidly. Considerations specific to the medical management of non-Alzheimer's dementia as it is pertinent to the nursing care of people with dementia are summarized in Table 4.2.

Chapter 4 Medical Management of Dementia

Table 4.2

Nursing Considerations Related to Medications for Non-Alzheimer's Dementia

Considerations for Non-Alzheimer's Dementia	Nursing Implications
Lewy body dementia increases sensitivity to adverse and therapeutic effects of many medications. Example: Risperidone and olanzapine are associated with higher incidence or exacerbation of extrapyramidal effects.	Use antipsychotics and benzodiazepines with caution. Use very low doses. Observe for adverse effects. If antipsychotics are necessary, quetiapine is the preferred drug. Teach about avoiding prescription and nonprescription products with strong anticholinergic properties, including decongestants and antihistamines. Assess for and document drug allergies and precautions.
People with Lewy body dementia may decompensate more when they have medical conditions.	Assess for physiological disorders as soon as behavior changes are observed.
Even during mild stages, Lewy body dementia causes autonomic nervous system dysfunctions affecting swallowing, digestion, blood pressure, temperature regulation, and bowel and bladder control.	Carefully assess all aspects of functioning. Teach about the importance of appropriate and consistent medical management by a neurologist or other specialist.
Movement and balance disorders often occur early in Lewy body dementia.	Facilitate referrals for physical and occupational therapy to promote safe and optimal functioning.
Risk factors associated with vascular dementia should be addressed early and consistently, especially during mild and moderate stages.	Teach patients and care partners to talk with primary care practitioners about management of cardiovascular risk factors, including lipids, blood pressure, and low-dose aspirin.

NONPRESCRIPTION AGENTS

As interest in complementary and integrative health has grown during the past two decades, there has been increasing emphasis on improving cognitive function through nonprescription agents such as herbs and vitamins. Healthcare professionals often are asked about these products, which are extensively marketed as beneficial not only for people with dementia, but also for all older adults. *Ginkgo biloba* and curcumin (turmeric) are herbs that may be neuroprotective in people with dementia; however, there is **little or no evidence-based support for other herbs or nonprescription products**. Nurses have important roles in teaching about nonprescription products for dementia because advertisements may not accurately reflect the most recent evidence-based information. In general, obtain information about the safety and efficacy of a product through reliable sources such as the National Center for Complementary and Integrative Health or the Food and Drug Administration as listed in the Resources. Additional points to include when teaching about nonprescription agents are as follows:

- Herbs and all other biologically active products can have adverse effects as well as drug interactions.
- Be sure to talk with your primary care practitioner about any nonprescription products you are using or considering using for health-related purposes.
- Because dietary supplements are not regulated, products vary in quality and do not necessarily contain the advertised quantity of ingredients.
- Dietary supplements do not have standardized quantities of ingredients, so an accurate dose is difficult to determine.

Fast Facts

Nurses have many opportunities to teach about nonprescription products for dementia.

◑ Clinical Snapshot

Mr. N, who is in the hospital for hip surgery, was recently diagnosed with dementia. When you are administering his donepezil he says, "I've been taking this medicine for 6 months and I don't seem to be any better. My wife says that I should start taking Ginkgo, do you know anything about that?" You respond, "Although some studies indicate that Ginkgo may be helpful, it's important to talk with your primary care practitioner about this and to be aware of drug interactions if you do take it. Also, it's important to obtain it from a reliable source because the quality of those products varies."

MEDICATIONS FOR MANAGEMENT OF DEMENTIA-RELATED SYMPTOMS

Medications are used for their direct effects on dementia and less commonly for the management of dementia-associated behaviors (as discussed extensively in Chapter 10, Emotional Needs of People With Dementia and Their Care Partners). Despite concerns about using behavior-modifying medications for people with dementia, **antipsychotics and antianxiety agents are sometimes necessary**, especially in acute care settings. If these medications are deemed necessary, follow these guidelines:

- Use the lowest effective dose.
- Establish clear nursing criteria for using PRN (as needed) medications (i.e., use only for patient safety or comfort, rather than for behaviors that are simply annoying).
- Frequently assess and document effects of medication.
- Assess for adverse effects, especially those that affect safety (e.g., increased fall risk, increased confusion).
- Assess optimal interval for administering PRN medications.
- Frequently reassess the need for medications.
- If antianxiety or antipsychotic medications have been initiated in an acute care setting, provide information in discharge documents, including instructions for follow-up as appropriate (including considerations for not continuing after discharge).

NONPHARMACOLOGIC INTERVENTIONS

Because there have been no major advances in the use of antidementia drugs since 2003, and there is **increasing concern about adverse effects of medications with anticholinergic effects,** the focus of **management has shifted to the use of nonpharmacologic interventions** for dementia-associated behaviors and issues. Chapters in Parts II through V provide a detailed discussion of interventions to address dementia-associated behaviors and issues related to safety and quality of life for people with dementia. In brief, nurses caring for people with dementia as a secondary diagnosis can incorporate the following interventions to address cognitive deficits in their usual course of providing care:

- State your name when you initiate communication.
- Make frequent casual references to the time of day, season of year, and so forth.
- Make sure information on dry-erase boards in patient rooms is accurate and up to date.
- Use simple written reminders about procedures and other scheduled activities.
- Provide frequent reminders about using the call system for assistance.
- Ask about pleasant memories and enjoyable activities (e.g., "Do you have a favorite memory about where you grew up?").
- Encourage use of simple relaxation practices (e.g., deep breathing, music).

Nurses can keep up to date on developments related to management of dementia by finding information from sites listed in the Resources section.

References

Jin, B.-R., & Liu, H-Y. (2019). Comparative efficacy and safety of cognitive enhancers for treating vascular cognitive impairment: Systematic review and Bayesian network meta-analysis. *Neural Regeneration Research, 14*(5), 805–816. doi:10.403/1673-5374.249228

Li, D-D., Zhang, Y-H., Zhang, W., & Zhao, P. (2019). Meta-analysis of randomized controlled trials on the efficacy and safety of donepezil, galantamine, rivastigmine, and memantine for the treatment of Alzheimer's disease. *Frontiers in Neuroscience, 13*, 472. doi:10.3389/fnins.219.00472

Logroscino, G., Imbimbo, B. P., Lozupone, M., Sardone, R., Capozzo, R., Battista, P., & Panza, F. (2019). Promising therapies for the treatment of frontotemporal dementia clinical phenotypes: From symptomatic to disease-modifying drugs. *Expert Opinions on Pharmacotherapy, 20*(9), 1091–1107. doi:10.1080/14656566.2019.159837

Meng, Y-H., Wang, P-P., Song, Y-X., & Wang, J-H. (2019). Cholinesterase inhibitors and memantine for Parkinson's disease dementia and Lewy body dementia: A meta-analysis. *Experimental and Therapeutic Medicine, 17,* 1611–1624. doi:10.3892/etm.2018.7129

Young, J. J., Lavakumar, M., Tampi, D., Balachandran, S., & Tampi, R. R. (2018). Frontotemporal dementia: Latest evidence and clinical implications. *Therapeutic Advances in Psychopharmacology, 8*(1), 33–41. doi:10.1177/2045125317739818

RESOURCES

Alzheimer's Association

https://www.alz.org

- Information about treatments and research

National Center for Complementary and Integrative Health

https://nccih.nih.gov/health/alzheimer

- Information about nonprescription treatments for dementia

Food and Drug Administration

*https://www.fda.gov/consumers/health-fraud-scams/unproven-alzheimers
    -disease-products*

- Information about unproven products for dementia

II

Person-Centered Care

5

Person-Centered Care for People With Dementia

INTRODUCTION

The current approach to caring for people with dementia emphasizes person-centered care that focuses on interventions to promote comfort and maintain the best quality of life for people with dementia and their families and care partners. This chapter discusses principles of person-centered care and identifies ways in which nurses can provide care that extends beyond the usual medical model to address issues related to the physical, mental, emotional, and spiritual needs of persons with dementia and their care partners.

In this chapter, you will learn:

1. Characteristics of person-centered care
2. Experiences of people with dementia
3. Providing culturally appropriate care

CHARACTERISTICS OF PERSON-CENTERED CARE

The term *person-centered care* has been used since the late 1990s to distinguish an approach to care for people with dementia that **emphasizes communication and relationship** from medical or behavioral approaches (Fazio, Pace, Flinner, & Kallmyer, 2018). Tom Kitwood, a British gerontologist, promulgated a model of person-centered care that has become widely accepted as a standard of care. Key concepts of this model include:

- The person being cared for is the center of all actions and decisions.
- Care is focused on the whole person, not just on the diagnosis, symptoms, or physical functioning.
- Interventions are directed toward maintaining and promoting comfort, dignity, respect, and a sense of wellness.
- Care plans emphasize strengths and abilities rather than deficits.
- Level of assistance is based on an assessment of the person's needs and abilities (i.e., not too much, not too little).
- Care plans identify and address emotional needs and personal preferences.
- Care settings are designed to promote positive social environments.
- The institutional environment needs to be adapted to compensate for the needs of people with dementia.

Although Kitwood's model was developed specifically for long-term care of people with dementia, the principles apply in any care setting. Exhibit 5.1 summarizes key points of this model as adopted in the Alzheimer's Association's practice recommendations.

Exhibit 5.1

Practice Recommendations for Person-Centered Care

Know the person living with dementia:

- Recognize that the individual with dementia is more than a diagnosis.
- Know the person's past and present unique values, beliefs, interests, abilities, likes, and dislikes.
- Use this information to inform every interaction and experience.

Recognize and accept the person's reality:

- See the world from the perspective of the person living with dementia.
- Recognize behavior as a form of communication.
- Promote effective and empathetic communication that validates feelings and connects the individual with his or her reality.

Identify and support ongoing opportunities for meaningful engagement:

- View every experience and interaction as an opportunity for engagement.

- Assure that engagement is meaningful to, and purposeful for, the individual living with dementia.
- Support the individual's interests and preferences.
- Allow for choice and success.
- Recognize that even when the dementia is most severe, the person can experience joy, comfort, and meaning in life.

Build and nurture authentic, caring relationships:

- Promote relationships that treat the individual with dignity and respect.
- Focus on presence.
- Concentrate on the interaction rather than the task.
- Emphasize "doing with" rather than "doing for."

Source: Fazio, S., Pace, D., Flinner, J., & Kallmyer, B. (2018). The fundamentals of person-centered care for individuals with dementia. *The Gerontologist, 58*, S10–S19. doi:10.1093/geront/gnx122. Used with permission.

Fast Facts

Incorporate information about likes and dislikes into care plans to facilitate care of people with dementia.

Clinical Snapshot

When Mrs. H, who has moderate dementia, is admitted for pneumonia, her daughter says she has difficulty chewing meat and hates the usual mechanical soft diet. You ask about food preferences and document that she enjoys casserole-type foods and will always eat sandwiches made with smooth peanut butter and jelly.

EXPERIENCES OF PEOPLE WITH DEMENTIA

In the words of a person with dementia:

If you are diagnosed with dementia, to others it sounds like, all of a sudden you are assumed to be incapable of anything. But actually, that's ridiculous.... You know, I have lots of experience, and that's not all gone at once. (van Wijngaarden, Alma, & The, 2019, p. 10)

A key component of providing person-centered care is to **understand how people with dementia experience and respond to their condition**. Imagine you have just arrived in a foreign country where you do not understand the language or recognize any of the people. This analogy illustrates that people with dementia may not understand verbal or written instructions, but they will notice nonverbal communication and interpret it in their unique ways. Talk with people who have mild and moderate dementia about their feelings and experiences, as discussed in Chapter 6, Communicating With People Who Have Dementia, and Chapter 7, Nursing Interventions for Early-Stage Dementia.

Nurses can ask simple questions such as, "So what techniques do you use to cope with your memory problems?" This emphasizes dementia as a chronic condition requiring coping skills. Moreover, it provides an opportunity to elicit information about the person's experience so you can identify and address their needs and feelings.

Fast Facts

There are many opportunities to identify and address the needs and feelings of people with dementia during the usual course of providing care.

Clinical Snapshot

During the admission assessment, Mrs. C tells you that she uses the rivastigmine (Exelon) patch because she was recently diagnosed with dementia. In response to your question about how she copes, she says, "Sometimes I feel pretty lonely and stupid because my bridge group doesn't want me there anymore and I used to have lunch and cards with them every week." You respond, "I'm sure it's hard to deal with dementia, and I appreciate you talking about your experiences. Did you know that the Alzheimer's Association has social, support, and educational programs for people with dementia? I can give you their phone number so you can call them after you get home."

PROVIDING CULTURALLY APPROPRIATE CARE

Person-centered care inherently recognizes and addresses the multidimensional cultural aspects that influence people with dementia and their care partners. Cultural background includes a wide range of characteristics, including race, ethnicity, religion, education, socioeconomic status, sexual orientation, sexual identity, and other sociocultural factors. These factors are likely to influence all the following aspects of care for people with dementia:

- Assessment of mental status
- Perceptions of cognitive changes
- Interpretation of dementia-related behaviors
- Beliefs about causes of mental changes
- Expectations related to caregiver roles within the family
- Acceptance of caregiver resources from outside the family
- Verbal communication (e.g., primary and secondary languages spoken and comprehended, which can change or fluctuate during the course of dementia)
- Nonverbal communication (e.g., touch, personal space, eye contact, facial expressions)
- Discussions about treatment options, including care during advanced dementia
- Management of pain and other symptoms
- Attitudes toward healthcare decisions (e.g., informed consent, healthcare proxies, advance directives)
- Acceptance of referrals for hospice, palliative care, and support services for the person with dementia and his or her care partners
- Acceptance of different healthcare practices, including use and acceptance of pharmacological and nonpharmacological interventions
- Use of various healthcare practitioners (e.g., physicians, nurse practitioners, herbalists, and complementary and alternative practitioners)

This book highlights cultural considerations related to specific aspects of care to increase awareness of different cultural perspectives. These considerations cannot be universally applied to any individual or particular group, but they provide a glimpse into diverse perspectives that may differ from the nurse's personal cultural viewpoint. Avoid stereotypes and generalizations and identify each person's unique perspective to provide culturally appropriate care. The resources at the end of this chapter list organizations that provide culturally specific health education materials in various languages.

Fast Facts

There are many opportunities to incorporate culturally appropriate interventions as an integral part of person-centered care for people with dementia and their families.

⟳ Clinical Snapshot

Mrs. S's daughter confides that she is overwhelmed with caring for her mother, who lives with her and has advanced dementia. Her mother was born in Puerto Rico and used to speak English, but now she understands only Spanish. You arrange for the hospital social worker to talk with her about local resources of the Alzheimer's Association, which provides culturally specific services for Hispanics.

References

Fazio, S., Pace, D., Flinner, J., & Kallmyer, B. (2018). The fundamentals of person-centered care for individuals with dementia. *The Gerontologist, 58*, S10–S19. doi:10.1093/geront/gnx122

Van Wijngaarden, E., Alma, M., & The, A-M. (2019). "The eyes of others" are what really matters: The experience of living with dementia from an insider perspective. *PLoS One, 14*(4), e0214724. doi:10.1371/journal.pone.0214724

RESOURCES

Long-Term Care Facilities That Incorporate Person-Centered Care

Advancing Excellence in America's Nursing Homes

https://qioprogram.org/nursing-home-resources/

• Information about national campaign to improve dementia care in nursing homes

Pioneer Network

https://www.pioneernetwork.net

• Information about person-centered care in nursing facilities

Dementia Information in Other Languages

Alzheimer's Disease International

https://www.alz.co.uk/other-languages

MedlinePlus

https://www.nlm.nih.gov/medlineplus/languages/dementia.html

6

Communicating With People Who Have Dementia

INTRODUCTION

Because dementia affects all aspects of communication through-out the course of the condition, nurses need to frequently assess communication difficulties and identify effective ways of com-municating verbally and nonverbally. When caring for people with dementia, the nurse's communication techniques often serve as an intervention not only for providing information in a way they can understand but also for addressing their psycho-social needs related to anxiety, distress, and emotional support.

In this chapter, you will learn:

1. Common communication issues during early-stage dementia
2. Common communication issues during moderate and advanced dementia
3. Nursing strategies for communicating with people with dementia
4. Nonverbal communication
5. Cultural considerations
6. Linguistic competence

COMMON COMMUNICATION ISSUES DURING EARLY-STAGE DEMENTIA

In the words of a person with dementia:

> I used to engage in conversations with other people but now I some-times notice that I don't give the right answers, you know, stray from the theme. That makes me terribly insecure. . . . Right now, I am scrutinizing my choice of words, but still I say crazy things. It makes me think, *You stupid fool!* I have this annoying feeling that I'm not equal anymore. (Van Wijngaarden, Alma, & The, 2019, p. 9)

Verbal communication is often one of the first aspects of func-tioning affected by dementia-related brain changes; in some cases, verbal abilities are affected months or even years before memory deficits. As dementia progresses, the person's ability to communicate verbally (i.e., expressive abilities) diminishes gradually until it even-tually becomes severely compromised during the advanced stage. Similarly, the person's ability to understand verbal communica-tion (i.e., receptive abilities) usually diminishes gradually. During all stages, **people with dementia may be able to understand non-verbal communication** but have difficulty understanding verbal communication.

Examples of Communication Difficulties

- Mispronunciation
- Inaccurate use of words
- Inability to finish sentences
- Difficulty finding the right word ("it's on the tip of my tongue but it can't come out")
- Using a general word when asked to name an item (*thing* instead of *pen*)
- Inability to follow complex discussions
- Difficulty communicating when the environment is noisy or otherwise distracting

In these situations, people with dementia and their families and care partners may benefit from **speech therapy services** to learn about techniques to facilitate communication. This is an aspect of care that is often overlooked, even though people with mild or moder-ate dementia can learn about techniques to improve communication. This is particularly important when families and care partners are motivated to learn how to facilitate communication between them-selves and the person with dementia.

Fast Facts

Communication disorders during mild and moderate dementia are complex. Consider making a referral for speech therapy to assist in developing a plan to improve communication.

Clinical Snapshot

Mrs. T has mild dementia and has been admitted for pneumonia. During her hospitalization, you assess that she has significant difficulty with word finding, but she tries very hard to communicate and becomes anxious when others do not understand her. When you discuss discharge plans with Mrs. T and her daughter, you suggest that they talk with her doctor about a referral for speech therapy because she has never been evaluated or taught about communication techniques for expressive aphasia.

In the words of a person with dementia:

> The daily communication with my partner is becoming a problem. To put it like this: if you draw two lines, her line continues on the same level, but mine deflects in a downward curve. Clearly our communication no longer runs in two parallel lines. As a result, I tend to withdraw. . . . More than before, I hesitate to ask or discuss things with her. That's a rotten side effect of dementia. (Van Wijngaarden et al., 2019, p. 12)

COMMON COMMUNICATION ISSUES DURING MODERATE AND ADVANCED DEMENTIA

Dementia gradually affects all aspects of verbal and nonverbal communication. Even in the most advanced stages, however, **assume the person retains some understanding of verbal and nonverbal messages** that we communicate. During moderate and advanced dementia, the following communication difficulties occur:

- Repetitious use of phrases, words, or sounds
- Misinterpretation of verbal and nonverbal communication
- Inability remembering recent events, but retained ability to talk about familiar experiences of childhood and earlier adulthood

- Increased difficulty understanding written or verbal communication, progressing to total inability
- Increased difficulty understanding nonverbal communication, but not to the point of total inability
- Reversion to the language used during childhood and younger adulthood or a mix of languages if English is a second language

Fast Facts

Dementia gradually affects all communication abilities, but even during advanced dementia, people are able to perceive messages that are communicated.

☼ Clinical Snapshot

Mrs. H, who has advanced dementia, repeatedly cries, "Help me, help me, I need to see her, I need to see her," when she is alone. When she is in a wheelchair near the nurses' station, she is quiet and less anxious because nurses and other staff frequently stop to touch her arm and reassure her that her daughter is coming soon.

NURSING STRATEGIES FOR COMMUNICATING WITH PEOPLE WITH DEMENTIA

Verbal Communication

Nurses routinely adapt their level of communication to the abilities of their patients, but this is very challenging when caring for people with dementia. **Ask families and care partners about helpful communication techniques** used prior to hospitalization so these can be incorporated in the care plan. People with mild dementia may be able to tell you what techniques improve their ability to communicate.

Guidelines for communicating with people with dementia:

- Avoid oversimplification for people with mild dementia. Use simpler sentences for people with moderate or advanced dementia.
- Assess the person's response to your communication by observing their verbal and nonverbal responses.

- Document effective and ineffective communication techniques in the care plan.
- Do not talk about a person with dementia as if they are not present.
- Assess the ability of the person with dementia to be included in discussions related to their care and include them appropriately.
- When discussions are about—rather than with—someone with dementia, hold these conversations out of hearing range of the person who is being talked about.
- If the person's hearing is impaired, make sure hearing aids are in place and functional, and use effective communication techniques.
- If the person has eyeglasses, make sure they are clean and being used.
- Accept that you may hear the same story repeatedly and this is okay.
- Involve a speech/language therapist for evaluation and management.

Table 6.1 lists examples of specific communication techniques that may be helpful for people with dementia.

Table 6.1

Techniques for Communicating With People With Dementia	
Communication Technique	Example
Allow time for processing.	Silently count to 10 after asking a question.
Use positive statements for directions.	Rather than stating "Don't get out of bed without help," say "Please call for help when you need to get out of bed."
Identify key words that the person uses in reference to activities.	A person with dementia says "gotta, gotta, gotta" when she needs to be directed to the bathroom.
Avoid statements that may be interpreted as judgmental.	Rather than stating "You need a bath today," say "It's time for your bath."
Rephrase statements that may be interpreted as placing the "blame" on the person with dementia.	Instead of stating "Your words are all so jumbled, you don't make any sense," say "I'm having trouble understanding your words. Can you try another word?"
Paraphrase or use other words if the person does not understand the first communication.	If the person does not comprehend "Tomorrow you'll be transferred to Sunny View Healthcare Center," say "Tomorrow you're going to another place for more therapy."

(*continued*)

Table 6.1

Techniques for Communicating With People With Dementia (*continued*)

Communication Technique	Example
Assist with word finding and clarify questionable words.	In response to "I don't know what my homework is?" (from a person with moderate dementia after returning from an x-ray), say "Are you wanting to know about the test you just had?"
Do not ask questions that you know the person cannot answer, but give clues to the correct information.	If a patient has not been able to state the name of the hospital, incorporate that information during usual conversations (e.g., "Is your daughter coming today to see you here at Centerville Hospital?")
Provide visual cues with accurate information.	Keep dry erase boards up to date; make sure clocks and watches are set for correct time.
Involve the person in decisions to the best of his or her ability by offering simple and concrete choices.	Say "Do you want chicken or steak?" rather than "What do you want to eat?"
Be specific and give one command at a time if the person can follow only one step at a time.	Separate commands, with time between them to perform each step: "Pick up this toothbrush . . . lift it to your mouth . . . brush your teeth."
Do not argue with or correct the person unless it is a matter of safety.	If the person tells you he is going to the ballgame this afternoon, but you know this is not true, do not challenge his statement unless he tries to leave.
Try to identify and respond to the person's feelings rather than simply stating facts.	If the person says her mother must be very busy because she has not visited today (and you know her mother is deceased), say "You must be missing her. What is a favorite memory of things you used to do with her?"
Use clues in the person's environment to initiate positive communication.	If you see flowers with a card, say something like "These are beautiful flowers from your daughter and her family. They must love you a lot."

Fast Facts

Nurses can assess patient communication patterns and adapt communication techniques to meet the needs of the person with dementia.

🔄 Clinical Snapshot

The care plan for Mrs. A, who has moderate dementia, incorporates the following interventions, based on the nursing assessment:
Provide bedpan when patient says "potty, potty, potty"; ask about two simple choices for liquid nourishment and meal selection; make sure Mrs. A has hearing aid in place when discussing care issues.

Many people, including nurses, are inclined to "talk down" to people who are cognitively impaired or physically disabled. This style of communication—sometimes called **elderspeak**—is disrespectful because it reflects a manner that is not generally used for adults. To avoid elderspeak, **pay attention to your tone of voice and inflection,** and use the same communication style as with adults who are not impaired. Another communication habit that can be perceived as disrespectful is the inaccurate use of plural pronouns when addressing an individual, as in "It's time to take our pills" or "How are we feeling today?" Even terms that are viewed as endearing, such as *honey* or *dearie*, are inappropriate when used for adults in care settings. Nurses and all care partners for people with dementia need to self-assess their communication patterns and edit any terms that are associated with infants, children, or one's loss of control over their own decisions. Table 6.2 lists examples of these kinds of terms along with appropriate alternatives that can be applied to communication with all older adults.

Fast Facts

Nurses communicate respect for people with dementia by avoiding the use of words that are associated with dependency or loss of decision-making abilities.

🔄 Clinical Snapshot

Mrs. V's son says, "I sure dread having to put her in a nursing home." You respond with, "It would be a good idea to look at the many places where she could be admitted for the care she requires. There are some very good dementia-care facilities that support the person's dignity and best level of functioning."

Table 6.2

Communicating Respectfully With Older Adults

Terms to Avoid	Respectful Terms
Diaper	Brief, incontinence product
Bib	Clothing protector
Feeding	Dining, eating, meals
Caretaker, caregiver	Helper, companion, assistant
Nursing home	Care facility, rehab center, skilled care center
Day care	Day center, day program
Nursing home "placement" or "putting in" a nursing home	Admitting for long-term care, or skilled nursing, or rehabilitation

Nonverbal Communication

As dementia progresses to moderate and advanced stages, **nonverbal communication becomes increasingly important**. This holds true for messages being sent both to and from the person with dementia. Pay close attention to what you communicate nonverbally—even unintentionally—as well as what the person with dementia is attempting to communicate.

Guidelines for nonverbal communication during moderate and advanced dementia:

- Assume that all nonverbal expressions of the person with dementia are attempts to communicate needs or feelings.
- Closely observe all nonverbal cues exhibited by the person, especially those that express feelings.
- Assume that even in advanced dementia, the person will perceive and understand nonverbal communication, such as touch.
- Be aware of your own nonverbal communication during all interactions, even when the person with dementia is observing you from a distance.
- Assume that your nonverbal cues will communicate more than your spoken words, and will be interpreted from the perspective of the person with dementia.

Table 6.3 provides example of nonverbal communication techniques that nurses can use for people with dementia.

Table 6.3

Nonverbal Communication Techniques When Caring for People With Dementia

Nonverbal Communication Technique	Example
Attract the person's attention before speaking.	Use direct eye contact or appropriate touching.
Pay attention to your facial expressions.	Use relaxed, smiling expressions; avoid expressions of anxiety or frustration.
Reinforce verbal communication with nonverbal communication that is consistent with your message.	When you want someone with moderate dementia to comb his hair, put the comb in his hand and mimic combing your hair.
Find out how the person responds to touch and use it appropriately.	Use gentle touch to gain the person's attention or reinforce feelings of concern, unless the person responds negatively to being touched.
Be aware of possible misinterpretation of your body language.	Avoid facial expressions or arm positions that communicate disapproval, such as scowling, wrinkled eyebrows, arms folded across chest, or arms out and on both hips.

Fast Facts

Nurses can use nonverbal communication purposefully when caring for people with dementia.

◔ Clinical Snapshot

When administering medications to Mr. R, who has moderate dementia, stand face-to-face, establish eye contact, place a cup of water in one of his hands, and ask him to open his other hand. After putting pills in his hand, demonstrate that he is to put the pills into his mouth and then drink the water.

CULTURAL CONSIDERATIONS

Cultural norms often hold a subtle but strong influence on nonverbal communication in any of the following ways:

- Cultural norms may influence the social acceptability of physical contact, particularly between men and women.

- Cultural backgrounds may influence the way a person uses facial expressions to communicate pain, happiness, or displeasure.
- Cultural groups hold differing social norms for physical touch, including hand shaking, with variations according to gender or age differences.
- Eye contact may be perceived according to social norms, with some groups considering direct eye contact as impolite, particularly between men and women.

People with dementia may become disinhibited in expressions of touch, or they may become more reluctant to be touched.

LINGUISTIC COMPETENCE

Person-centered care involves linguistic competence (i.e., communication that is respectful of and responsive to a person's linguistic needs) for people who do not speak English as a primary language. For people with dementia, even if they learned English as a second language, they are likely to have **better communication in their native language as their condition progresses**. Since 2001, all healthcare institutions that receive federal funds are required to provide access to 24-hour, no-cost language assistance for individuals who need it. Nurses may need to initiate a request for such a service to improve communication and provide culturally appropriate care.

Reference

Van Wijngaarden, E., Alma, M., & The, A-M. (2019). "The eyes of others" are what really matters: The experience of living with dementia from an insider perspective. *PLoS One, 14*(4), e0214724. doi:10.1371/journal.pone.0214724

RESOURCES

Hartford Institute for Geriatric Nursing

https://consultgerirn.org
- Communication difficulties: Assessment and interventions in hospitalized older adults with dementia, *Try This*, Issue D7, article and video

Tips on communication issues related to dementia

- *https://alz.org/help-support/caregiving/daily-care/communications*
- *https://alz.org/national/documents/brochure_communication.pdf*
- *https://www.nia.nih.gov/health/alzheimers-caregiving-changes-communication-skills*
- *https://www.nhs.uk/conditions/dementia/communication-and-dementia*

III

Nursing Considerations for People With Dementia During Specific Stages

7

Nursing Interventions for Early-Stage Dementia

INTRODUCTION

The diagnosis of dementia is based on a comprehensive evaluation of cognitive and personality changes that have developed over years, except in the relatively few cases when a stroke or other major medical event causes acute changes. Manifestations of early-stage dementia occur gradually, and only the person with dementia and his or her close contacts notice the changes. During this stage, people with dementia can maintain a relatively safe and independent level of functioning, but they need to compensate for cognitive deficits. They may be able to live alone with help from support resources, or they may be living with their spouse or family or in an assisted living facility.

Nurses can recognize early-stage dementia under any of the following circumstances:

- *The person or care partner reports cognitive impairments that interfere significantly with daily functioning and have been occurring during the previous months or years.*
- *Nurses observe significant cognitive impairments that are not associated with another diagnosis (e.g., delirium, depression).*
- *A diagnosis of dementia has been documented, and the person is functioning at a relatively independent level.*

In either of the first two circumstances, nursing responsibilities focus on assessment issues, and in all circumstances, nurses caring for people with early-stage dementia focus on issues related to both safety and quality of life.

In this chapter, you will learn:

1. Characteristics of early-stage dementia
2. Assessment issues and related nursing strategies
3. Cultural considerations
4. Safe and independent functioning
5. Quality-of-life issues

CHARACTERISTICS OF EARLY-STAGE DEMENTIA

In the words of a person with dementia:

> People often think that anyone in early stage couldn't possibly have dementia because their vision of dementia is only about end stage. . . . The sooner we can change public perception the better it will be for all of us living with dementia. We don't start out at that stage and some of us take a LONG time until we get there. (Kannaley, Mehta, Yelton, & Friedman, 2019, p. 9)

The **early-stage dementia** of the Alzheimer's type is characterized by the following changes that occur gradually and are experienced by the person with dementia and noticed by people who are in close contact with the person:

- Impaired short-term memory for names, events, appointments, and other information
- Difficulty performing familiar tasks in social or work situations
- Difficulty recalling information that was just read or heard
- Frequently misplacing or losing important objects
- Diminished ability to plan or organize tasks

If significant personality or behavioral changes also occur during the early stage, the type of dementia may be Lewy body, or frontotemporal. If the changes occur episodically with periodic improvements, the type of dementia may be vascular. When dementia is a non-Alzheimer's type, the person's memory and other cognitive characteristics may not be affected during the early stage. Because of the difficulty in distinguishing between types of dementia during the early stage, obtain information about the onset and progression of various characteristics for the diagnostic process.

ASSESSMENT ISSUES AND RELATED NURSING STRATEGIES

In the words of a person with dementia:

> I have to cover up, you know. Well, say I'm in a conversation with somebody and I have to admit to them either that I have lost the plot completely or something disturbed me, or something. I have to find an excuse for not getting it right. (Xanthopoulou & McCabe, 2019, p. 5)

Some people with dementia are acutely aware of the earliest changes, whereas **others have little or no insight or awareness** during the course of this condition. Some patients will offer information about having dementia, while others will adamantly insist that they have no cognitive impairments despite evidence to the contrary. People with early-stage dementia may object to obtaining an evaluation, but this does not mean that such a discussion should be avoided. Rather, address the issue in a similar manner to suggesting an assessment of other aspects of functioning. Ask patients or their families and care partners about any evaluation of cognitive or personality changes, and emphasize that a good assessment will help identify conditions that can be treated with the goal of improving or reversing the changes.

Fast Facts

During the course of usual nursing care, discuss observations about the person's memory (or other aspects of cognition) and ask if this has been addressed in any medical evaluation.

Clinical Snapshot

When you perform the initial nursing assessment on Mrs. T, who is being admitted for upper gastrointestinal (GI) bleeding, you note that she repeatedly asks the same questions and seems to give inaccurate information in response to your questions. You say, "I noticed that you have some trouble with your memory. Have you talked with your doctor about this so it can be evaluated?"

In some situations, **dementia may have been diagnosed but not documented** as a current problem—particularly when care is focused on acute conditions. If the person is taking a dementia-specific medication (as discussed in Chapter 4, Medical Management of Dementia), ask about the related diagnosis. Use Table 7.1 as a guide to addressing assessment issues commonly associated with early-stage dementia.

Table 7.1

Assessment Issues and Related Nursing Strategies	
Assessment Issues	**Nursing Strategies**
Different levels of awareness of cognitive impairments	Ask open-ended questions about changes in ability to remember things or manage usual responsibilities Assess whether the reported level of functioning is consistent with objective assessment findings.
Attributing significant changes to "normal aging"	Emphasize that there are many conditions that affect cognitive functioning for people at all ages and that it is important to identify those that can be treated.
Family members express concern about cognitive changes, but the person with early-stage dementia has no awareness of impairments or denies the need for assessment	Identify an aspect of functioning that the person acknowledges is problematic or talk with the person about the concerns noted by the family and encourage the person to have this evaluated so that treatable conditions can be identified.
Not enough time to address assessment issues	Document concerns and teach about the importance of having cognitive changes evaluated as part of the discharge plan.

Fast Facts

Many strategies can be used to facilitate an evaluation of people with manifestations of early-stage dementia (Table 7.1).

CULTURAL CONSIDERATIONS

In recent years, dementia has become a global health priority—a phenomenon largely attributable to the rapid and ongoing increase in the older adult population worldwide. Thus, dementia is now recognized as a "global health priority of our age" (Hillman & Latimer, 2017). Within a cross-cultural context, recognize that **the term dementia is a Western construct,** as is the designation of what is considered normal and abnormal aging (Sagbakken, Spilker, & Nielsen, 2018).

Examples of cultural variations related to the perception of dementia:

- Manifestations of what is considered "mental illness" as shameful; these changes are likely to be ignored, denied, or covered up.
- Memory impairment and other cognitive changes may be considered normal and acceptable signs of aging; there is no need to consider medical evaluation or treatment.
- In China, people with dementia may face ridicule and isolation and be referred to in terms such as "stupid, demented elderly" (Calia, Johnson, & Cristea, 2019).

SAFE AND INDEPENDENT FUNCTIONING

People with early-stage dementia typically live alone or with a spouse, partner, or family member and require some supervision or minimal assistance when performing complex activities.

Common safety concerns during early-stage dementia include driving, meal preparation, and accurate management of finances and medications. During the early stage, these concerns usually do not pose major threats; however, they are likely to present additional risks to safety as the dementia progresses.

Although inpatient settings may present limited opportunities to address safety issues related to home settings, **home safety risks can be addressed in discharge plans**. Nurses in acute care settings, including ED, need to assess whether cognitive impairments have contributed to the presenting problem. For example, early-stage dementia can compromise the ability to take medications accurately, and this may have led to the emergency medical condition (as described in the Clinical Snapshot at the end of this chapter). Nurses in community-based settings have opportunities to identify risks for safe functioning and teach about strategies to reduce the risk.

Safety concerns can be assessed by asking the person about any difficulties in performing daily activities and by obtaining information from family members and care partners. When safety concerns are noted, you can teach simple strategies to diminish the risk, as detailed in Table 7.2.

Fast Facts

Use assessment questions to identify "red flags" for potential safety concerns.

Clinical Snapshot

Mr. B's daughter tells you she is wondering if her father is safe living alone because he has dementia and he drives to church and the grocery store. You ask about all of the following: recent car accidents, dents in the car, burned pots and pans, ability to take medications as prescribed, ability to initiate phone calls if he needs help, and evidence of bills not being paid or money that cannot be accounted for.

Table 7.2

Safety Concerns and Related Nursing Strategies

Safety Concern	Nursing Strategies to Diminish the Risk
Questions about safe driving	Suggest that a formal driving evaluation be performed by a specially trained occupational therapist. Emphasize that the person may qualify for a driving rehabilitation program or may be safe with certain restrictions. Refer to the appropriate resources listed at the end of this chapter.
Difficulty managing medications	Teach about the many medication-management systems that can be used, ranging from readily available daily dosing containers to more complex automated 28-day systems. Refer to the appropriate resources listed at the end of this chapter.
Unsafe use of stove	Consider installing shutoff valves or removing knobs. Use an electric tea kettle with automatic shutoff for boiling water; encourage use of a microwave oven if this can be done safely.
Risk for financial exploitation; inability to manage bill paying	Teach about the importance of establishing a financial power of attorney and having a trustworthy person assist as necessary with financial management.

Fast Facts

In any clinical setting, nurses have opportunities to assess for or ask about safety concerns and suggest interventions (Table 7.2).

⚙ Clinical Snapshot

Mrs. T tells you she has been diagnosed with Alzheimer's disease, and now her friends do not want her in their bridge club. You respond, "I'm sure you have lots to offer in other ways because you are so friendly and have traveled a lot. Would you be willing to participate in the Memory Lane group that meets here every Wednesday afternoon after lunch?"

QUALITY-OF-LIFE ISSUES

People with early-stage dementia consistently express the need to be recognized as individuals and receive support from healthcare professionals to strengthen their coping abilities. In recent years, local chapters of the Alzheimer's Association, which are available in every community, have increasingly addressed the needs of people with early-stage dementia. As part of ongoing care or in discharge plans, suggest that people with early-stage dementia consider participating in support and educational groups, either in person or through online resources.

In the words of a person with dementia:

It's just a group of people who have also been told they have Alzheimer's. One is in a more advanced stage than the other, but I feel comfortable. We value and fully respect each other. We laugh, talk, drink coffee, and do nice things. (Van Wijngaarden, Alma, & The, 2019, p. 13)

At the minimum, **provide the phone number of the local Alzheimer's Association chapter** and encourage exploration of this resource. Explain that even if the person has not been diagnosed with Alzheimer's, this organization is an excellent source of information and provides support resources about cognitive impairments and all types of dementia. In addition, provide a copy of the Resources section at the end of this chapter and encourage people with dementia and their care partners to explore these resources.

Fast Facts

Nurses caring for people with early-stage dementia in any setting can ask them about their feelings and experiences, with emphasis on their ways of coping.

🌀 Clinical Snapshot: Nursing Care for a Person With Early-Stage Dementia in the ED

Mrs. S, a 78-year-old widow who lives alone, was brought to the ED after she passed out while playing cards with friends. She is alert and responsive and oriented x3. Her medications include furosemide (Lasix) every morning, ramipril (Altace) twice daily, metoprolol (Lopressor) twice daily, and potassium powder effervescent (Klor-Con/EF). All diagnostic tests are within normal, except for a serum potassium of 2.8 mEq/L. When you ask about her medications, she reports that she takes one water pill and two heart pills in the morning, and sometimes an extra water pill in the afternoon if her feet are swollen. Upon further questioning, she tells you that she thinks she's been taking the extra water pill recently, but she really cannot remember how often. You specifically ask about the potassium powder and she states, "Oh, I usually forget to take that because it's not in the compartment with my other pills." When Mrs. S's daughter arrives, you ask if she has noticed changes in her mother's cognitive abilities, and she reports that her mother has been forgetting appointments and has not been paying her bills as usual. The daughter has been concerned about these changes and considered having an evaluation at the geriatric assessment program. You teach Mrs. S and her daughter about the importance of following through with the geriatric assessment appointment, and you suggest that Mrs. S allow her daughter to oversee her medication system.

References

Calia, C., Johnson, H., & Cristea, M. (2019). Cross-cultural representations of dementia: An exploratory study. *Journal of Global Health, 9*(1), 011001. doi:10.7189/jogh.09.01.011001

Hillman, A., & Latimer, J. (2017). Cultural representations of dementia. *PLoS Medicine, 14*(3), e1002274. doi:10.1371/journal.pmed.1002274

Kannaley, K., Mehta, S., Yelton, B., & Friedman, D. B. (2019). Thematic analysis of blog narratives written by people with Alzheimer's disease and other dementias and care partners. *Dementia, 18*(7–8), 3071–3090. doi:10.1177/1471301218768162

Sagbakken, M., Spilker, P. S., & Nielsen, T. R. (2018). Dementia and immigrant groups: A qualitative study of challenges related to identifying, assessing, and diagnosing dementia. *BMC Health Services Research, 18*(1), 910. doi:10.1186/s12913-018-3720-7

Van Wijngaarden, E., Alma, M., & The, A-M. (2019). "The eyes of others" are what really matters: The experience of living with dementia from an insider perspective. *PLoS One, 14*(4), e0214724. doi:10.1371/journal.pone.0214724

Xanthopoulou, P., & McCabe, R. (2019). Subjective experiences of cognitive decline and receiving a diagnosis of dementia: Qualitative interviews with people recently diagnosed in memory clinics in the UK. *BMJ Open, 9*(8), e026071. doi:10.1035/bmjopen-2018-026071.

RESOURCES

Alzheimer's Association

https://www.alz.org

- Information about educational and support services for people with early-stage dementia and their families and care partners
- Information about medical alert devices specifically for people with dementia

Family Caregiver Alliance, National Center on Caregiving

https://www.caregiver.org

- Information about early-stage dementia

8

Moderate-Stage Dementia

INTRODUCTION

Moderate-stage dementia is best described as the stage between early and advanced dementia. There are no clear boundaries among any of the stages because, although dementia progresses gradually, the course is not necessarily a consistent downhill path. Rather, people with dementia fluctuate in their functioning because of changes in health status, environment, care partners, and other conditions. This chapter focuses on nursing issues that are most closely associated with moderate-stage dementia, but the information in most of the other chapters of the book is also pertinent to this stage of dementia.

In this chapter, you will learn:

1. Characteristics of moderate-stage dementia
2. Common issues during moderate-stage dementia
3. Cultural considerations
4. Referrals for assistance with decision-making
5. Safe and independent functioning

CHARACTERISTICS OF MODERATE-STAGE DEMENTIA

In the words of a person with dementia:

> I'm afraid I don't have a very positive message. Actually, I'm really suffering due to the influence of dementia. You know, I have a lot of problems with the growing distance between me and my relatives. . . . They just go on with their lives, and I cannot keep up with them any longer. I know it's just one of the consequences of dementia, this distance between you and the ones you love, but it makes me very sad. (van Wijngaarden, Alma, & The, 2019, p. 15)

Reisberg's (1986) widely used scale for **Functional Assessment of Alzheimer's Disease (FAST)** describes characteristics of moderate and moderately severe dementia as:

- Obvious cognitive deficits (e.g., disorientation, significant short-term memory impairment)
- Difficulty remembering names of familiar people
- Unable to manage complex daily tasks without supervision or assistance
- Gradual loss of ability to perform activities of daily living (dressing, bathing, toileting)
- Development of urinary incontinence
- Development of bowel incontinence

These changes usually develop slowly over several years or they may develop more rapidly if there are significant medical events, such as stroke or major surgery. In addition, a major change in support, such as loss of a significant care partner, can precipitate a rapid decline in functioning. In these situations, the person may seem to move rapidly from early- to moderate-stage dementia, but the ongoing dementia pathology may actually be stable.

Fast Facts

If a person with early-stage dementia seems to move quickly to the moderate stage, this may be due to a concomitant medical condition or to a major change in caregiver support.

⊙ **Clinical Snapshot**

After Mrs. C's husband of 56 years died, her children noted that she was easily confused, did not remember what day it was, did not take her daily medications, forgot to eat, did not bathe, and was unsafe living alone. When they assessed the situation, they realized that their father had provided so much supervision and assistance that her early dementia was well hidden. They also found out that she had been taking galantamine (Razadyne) but had not told them about this.

COMMON ISSUES DURING MODERATE-STAGE DEMENTIA

During moderate-stage dementia, both the person with dementia and their care partners need to adjust to the gradually increasing need for assistance with daily activities. **Decisions about living arrangements usually arise** for people with dementia who do not live with someone who can assume the necessary caregiving role. When the person lives with or depends on spouse or family, decisions about support for caregivers and use of outside resources are usually a major concern.

Situations often involve conflicts about independence versus safety or self-determination versus allowing others to make decisions. The process is particularly challenging when the person with dementia does not have the insight and capacity to make safe and reasonable choices. During this phase, families, care partners, and people with dementia often seek advice from nurses.

Assist with these decisions by using Exhibit 8.1 to assess aspects of functioning pertinent to decisions about care. Information in Chapter 7, Nursing Interventions for Early-Stage Dementia, particularly Table 7.2, can be used as a guide to assess safety concerns that arise during early dementia and continue through moderate-stage dementia. In addition, an important intervention is to **suggest or initiate referrals for assistance with complex decisions,** as discussed in the next section.

Exhibit 8.1

Assessment Issues and Related Nursing Actions

Cognitive abilities

- Use cognitive assessment tools (e.g., mini-mental status examination).
- Refer for geriatric assessment; assess memory, decision-making, and other cognitive functions during all interactions.
- Document all findings.

Emotional aspects

- Use screening tool for depression.
- Ask about feelings and coping skills related to dementia.
- Ask about spiritual/religious needs.

Ability to call for help

- Assess ability to use call light.
- Assess or ask care partners about ability to initiate phone calls unassisted.
- Assess ability to learn about emergency call system.

Personal care activities

- Assess grooming, bathing, oral care, and nail care.
- Refer for occupational therapy if appropriate.

Mobility

- Assess balance, walking, and transferring.
- Observe the person's interactions with the environment.
- Refer for physical therapy if appropriate.

Bowel and bladder control

- Assess for ongoing or intermittent urinary or fecal incontinence.
- Refer for evaluations as indicated (including checking for urinary tract infection).
- Assess for constipation or fecal impaction.
- Assess factors that increase the risk for incontinence (e.g., inaccessibility of toileting facility, relying on others for assistance).

Social supports

- Ask about changes in social contacts (e.g., are there enjoyable activities that you no longer do?).
- Ask about transportation limitations.

In addition, teach families and care partners about interventions to promote safe and independent functioning, as discussed in the last section of this chapter.

◐ Clinical Snapshot

You are caring for Ms. R, who has been admitted for knee replacement surgery and has dementia as a secondary diagnosis. Upon admission, her hair was greasy and unkempt, she had a strong body odor and bad breath, and her clothes were soiled. She told

(continued)

(continued)

you she lived alone and "I can take care of myself as I always have." You request an occupational therapy assessment and you arrange for the social worker to meet with Ms. R and her niece, who lives nearby and provides assistance with transportation and grocery shopping.

In the words of a person with dementia:

> I keep worrying you see in case I'm doing something.... How quickly will I get very noticeable? (Xanthopoulou & McCabe, 2019, p. 5)

CULTURAL CONSIDERATIONS

Family and societal expectations, often strongly influenced by cultural norms, play an influential role in decisions about care for the person with dementia. For example, in many cultures, families expect daughters will assume full caregiving roles and sons will provide financial support. In addition, expectations may be influenced by family caregiving history. For instance, conflict may arise if a widowed mother expects to move in with her daughter's family because her mother moved in with her family after her mother developed dementia. Nurses can **help alleviate stress associated with decision-making about care by suggesting referrals** as discussed in the subsequent section.

REFERRALS FOR ASSISTANCE WITH DECISION-MAKING

Nurses do not always have the skills or time to facilitate making decisions about care of people with dementia, but they can refer for social worker assistance. Nurses can also **suggest that families explore the wide range of caregiving resources and living arrangements**, including assisted living, senior apartments with additional services, and specialized dementia care facilities. In addition, provide contact information (see the Resources at the end of this chapter) for the following types of resources to assist with these decisions:

- Geriatric assessment programs for comprehensive multidisciplinary assessment and recommendations
- Geriatric care managers for initial and ongoing assistance with decisions about appropriate care
- Alzheimer's Association information hotline for advice about local resources
- Eldercare Locator for information about appropriate local resources

Emphasize that the increasing focus on person-centered care prompted the development of holistic models of care for people with dementia. Care partners can find information about facilities that provide person-centered care at the websites listed in the Resources section at the end of Chapter 5.

Fast Facts

Nurses can provide information about resources to assist with decisions about care issues, including conflicts related to safety versus independence.

🌀 **Clinical Snapshot**

Mr. P's son confides that he thinks his father should move to an assisted living facility, but his father will not discuss this because he is "fiercely independent and stubborn as well." You provide contact information of local geriatric assessment programs and care managers and urge him to call. You emphasize that staff in these programs are happy to discuss the situation and can arrange for an assessment and recommendations.

SAFE AND INDEPENDENT FUNCTIONING

Implement strategies to promote safe and independent functioning, for example by modifying environments and teaching families about interventions such as those summarized in Exhibit 8.2.

Exhibit 8.2

Nursing Actions to Promote Safe and Independent Functioning

Vision

- Plan for annual eye examinations.
- Maintain up-to-date prescription glasses.
- Keep eyeglasses clean.
- Provide optimal lighting.
- Ensure use of magnifying aids.

Hearing

- Plan for hearing evaluation.

- Ensure use of hearing aid or amplifying device.
- Assist as necessary with hearing aid care, insertion, and secure storage.
- Employ good communication techniques.

Memory and cognition

- Provide accurate information on orientation board.
- Ensure visibility of clocks and calendars.
- Place photos and other reminders of family and caring relationships in visible locations.

Personal care

- Provide reminders and assist as necessary, but allow as much independence as possible.
- Arrange for manicures, pedicures, and podiatry.
- Arrange personal care items in a visible and uncluttered place in the order in which they are used.
- Leave a toothbrush with toothpaste on it on the sink.

Mobility

- Ensure use of assistive devices as recommended.
- Arrange for physical therapy.
- Encourage participation in group exercise programs (including tai chi).
- Provide individual assistance for safety.

Bowel and bladder control

- Devise individualized toileting plan for maximum independence but with minimal risk for incontinence.
- Offer interventions to prevent constipation.

General safety and functioning

- Provide visual cues to designate important places (e.g., toilet, refrigerator).
- Provide simple cues for operating thermostats, appliances, radios, televisions, and so forth.

Usual environment

- Keep the environment simple and uncluttered.
- Keep medications, cleaning solutions, and any poisonous chemicals in inaccessible places.

Wayfinding difficulties

- Enroll in a protective program, such as the Safe Return program sponsored by the Alzheimer's Association.
- Teach about the importance of carrying identification.

Nurses have many opportunities to teach about interventions to promote safe and independent functioning.

⟳ Clinical Snapshot

You are caring for Mr. T after his cardiac surgery and observe that his eyeglasses look old and the side pieces are taped. He has a secondary diagnosis of dementia and lives in an assisted living facility. He cannot report information about his vision or eye examinations, but you assess that he cannot read the instructions about postsurgical care that were provided for him. When you meet with his daughter to discuss discharge plans, you find out that he has not had his eyes examined for at least 4 years. You emphasize that an annual eye examination is especially important for people with dementia because accurate sensory input is essential for compensating for cognitive deficits.

References

Reisberg, B. (1986). Dementia: A systematic approach to identifying reversible causes. *Geriatrics, 41*(4), 30–46.

Van Wijngaarden, E., Alma, M., & The, A-M. (2019). "The eyes of others" are what really matters: The experience of living with dementia from an insider perspective. *PLoS One, 14*(4), e0214724. doi:10.1371/journal.pone.0214724

Xanthopoulou, P., & McCabe, R. (2019). Subjective experiences of cognitive decline and receiving a diagnosis of dementia: Qualitative interviews with people recently diagnosed in memory clinics in the UK. *BMJ Open, 9*(8), e026071. doi:10.1035/bmjopen-2018-026071

RESOURCES

Alzheimer's Association

https://www.alz.org

- Resource for locating local service providers and support groups for people with dementia and their family

Eldercare Locator

https://www.eldercare.gov

- Excellent resource finding local services related to all aspects of care for people with dementia

9

Caring for the Person With Advanced Dementia

INTRODUCTION

Person-centered care focuses on comfort and quality of life for people with dementia and their care partners, and this focus becomes increasingly more important as dementia progresses. During the advanced phase, people with dementia have limited ability to express their needs and are no longer able to participate in decisions about care. Nurses have major roles in caring for people with advanced dementia and in supporting and advising care partners. This chapter focuses on nursing issues that are most closely associated with advanced dementia, but the information in many other chapters is also pertinent to this stage of dementia.

In this chapter, you will learn:

1. Characteristics of advanced dementia
2. Goals of treatment
3. Challenges related to nutrition
4. Supportive and end-of-life care
5. Cultural considerations
6. Nursing care for comfort

CHARACTERISTICS OF ADVANCED DEMENTIA

Dementia is a life-limiting condition and a leading cause of death, with the **advanced stage characterized by gradually increasing frailty and disability**. As with other stages of dementia, there is no line of demarcation indicating that the person has advanced dementia, and in the absence of acute medical conditions, the changes are usually subtle. Exhibit 9.1 describes some of the characteristics of advanced dementia.

Exhibit 9.1

Characteristics of Advanced Dementia

Cognition

- Unaware of surroundings
- Unable to recognize familiar people
- Severely impaired memory
- Severely impaired judgment and decision-making

Communication

- Extremely limited verbal communication
- Few intelligible words
- Unable to comprehend and follow instructions
- Eventually unable to smile
- Unable to verbally express needs or symptoms of pain or distress

Functional level

- Unable to perform activities of daily living, including eating, hygiene, toileting, and dressing
- Unsteady and deteriorating gait, eventually bedridden
- Unable to perform purposeful actions
- Eventually becomes totally incontinent of bladder and bowel

Sleep and activity level

- Shows little or no interest in activities
- Disrupted and inconsistent sleep patterns
- Eventually may sleep all or most of the time

Nutrition

- Loss of appetite, forgetting to eat
- Difficulty with chewing and swallowing
- Risk of aspiration
- Weight loss

Communication

- Loss of ability to verbally communicate
- Presumed awareness of emotions communicated by others
- May have heightened awareness of nonverbal communication from others
- Presumed nonverbal expressions of emotions and needs

Medical complications

- Increased incidence of seizures, pneumonia, dehydration, infection, electrolyte imbalances, and metabolic disturbances

Safety and behavioral concerns

- Unintentional self-harm caused by frequent falls or poor fluid and nutritional intake
- Nonaggressive agitation (e.g., repetitive vocalization, moaning, crying)

Fast Facts

Advanced dementia can last for months or years and is characterized by a gradual loss of all physical functioning and the ability to express needs.

GOALS OF TREATMENT

In the words of a person with dementia:

> When it comes to a worthy and dignified end of life, my keyword is self-determination. I want to end my life as a rational, sane person. At the moment, my thinking abilities are already a little compromised, have to admit, but I really want to stay in control till the end of my life. (Van Wijngaarden, Alma, & The, 2019, p. 17)

During all phases of dementia, goals of care focus on quality of life, but during the early and moderate phases, an additional focus is on curative and disease-modifying interventions for dementia as well as concomitant conditions. As dementia progresses, goals shift toward a primary focus on all the following aspects:

- Quality of life
- Optimal care environment
- Dignity and comfort
- Family support

- Maintenance of social connectedness
- Quality of death (McInerney, Doherty, Bindoff, Robinson, & Vickers, 2018)

This type of care, called **supportive or palliative care, is available through specialized dementia or palliative care programs**. People with advanced dementia are no longer able to participate in decisions about goals for their care, so families, healthcare proxies, and other care partners assume responsibility. If legal issues have been addressed during earlier stages, as discussed in Chapter 17, Ethical and Legal Issues, surrogate decision makers will have guidelines to follow. Even when advance directives are in place, surrogate decision makers and all care partners experience many emotional conflicts and ethical dilemmas because of the serious responsibility of implementing end-of-life wishes. Nurses have **essential roles in supporting surrogate decision makers**, and they can emphasize that the surrogate is acting out of love and concern by advocating for what the person with dementia wants.

Additional Roles of Nurses

- Providing nursing input in interdisciplinary teams to discuss clinical issues
- Providing information to caregivers about evidence-based guidelines for decisions
- Reviewing advance directives as the person's condition changes
- Assisting with discussions about implementation of advance directives
- Making referrals for social services, ethics committees, or other resources to address conflicts related to healthcare decisions and interventions
- Teaching caregivers about interventions for comfort
- Providing information about supportive, palliative, or hospice care
- Encouraging families and care partners to express their feelings and responding with compassion
- Suggesting referrals for caregiver support programs and other appropriate resources

Fast Facts

Communicating empathy for families and care partners who are dealing with challenging decisions about care of the person with advanced dementia is an important nursing intervention.

CHALLENGES RELATED TO NUTRITION

Feeding and eating difficulties usually begin during the middle stage of dementia and gradually worsen. Major care issues in advanced dementia include increased risks for aspiration, dehydration, weight loss, nutritional deficits, and aspiration pneumonia. Nurses, families, and care partners experience complex and powerful emotional and ethical concerns in addressing feeding and eating difficulties.

During the 1990s, percutaneous endoscopic gastrostomy (PEG) tubes were commonly used to provide fluid and nutrition to people with dementia. More recently, however, many questions have been raised about this practice because evidence does not support this intervention for people with advanced dementia. The current emphasis is on comfort feeding only as the best practice for addressing feeding and eating difficulties. This means that the person will not be forced to eat but will receive as much assistance as needed and will be fed so long as the process is not distressing.

Because people with advanced dementia cannot participate in complex decision-making, **families and care partners need accurate information about interventions for nutrition**, including the insertion of PEG tubes. Nurses can teach the following points when they discuss this with families and care partners:

- No evidence supports the use of feeding tubes as an effective intervention in people with advanced dementia.
- Feeding tubes are associated with complications (e.g., physical or pharmacological restraints and deprivation of the pleasure of food).
- Foregoing tube feeding does not mean the person's nutritional needs will be ignored.
- Comfort food is defined as any food that the person will accept, eat, and tolerate.
- Nursing and dietary staff will work with families and other care partners to identify the most appropriate and acceptable foods and fluids for the person with advanced dementia.
- Related interventions include providing meticulous oral care and using verbal and nonverbal communication that is comforting and encouraging during the feeding process.

Nurses are responsible for assuring that comfort feeding is carried out by staff. Nurses may need to arrange for more flexible and frequent mealtimes for patients with advanced dementia and plan these corresponding to the availability of someone who can take time for the hand-feeding process. In addition, nurses can initiate referrals for consultation from dieticians and speech-language therapists. These healthcare professionals are skilled in addressing issues related to nutrition and eating in people with dementia.

Fast Facts

Care providers address complex and emotional issues related to usual care issues such as food and fluids.

Clinical Snapshot

Mrs. V is admitted to the hospital with aspiration pneumonia. She resides in a nursing home and a swallowing evaluation indicates that she requires honey-thick foods. Mrs. V's daughter tells you that her mother does not like the thickened diet and she often finds cookies, crackers, and other snacks to eat in the drawers of other residents. You initiate referrals for a speech therapist and dietician to advise about foods that are safe and acceptable for Mrs. V.

SUPPORTIVE AND END-OF-LIFE CARE

A major challenge for families and care partners of people with advanced dementia is determining when the person moves into the terminal phase, which is generally defined as the 6 months prior to death. Of course, there is no crystal ball to predict the timeline, but consider the following factors in determining hospice eligibility based on an expected 6-month survival:

- Progressive loss of all verbal and psychomotor abilities (functional assessment staging 7)
- Dementia-related comorbidities: Sepsis, aspiration, persistent fever, upper urinary tract infection, multiple stage 3–4 pressure ulcers, and significant weight loss within 6 months
- Significant comorbidities: Cancer, congestive heart failure, unstable medical condition
- Additional considerations: Oxygen therapy needed, shortness of breath, less than 25% of food eaten at most meals, bowel incontinence, sleeping most of the time

When dementia progresses to the terminal phase, goals increasingly **focus on comfort and quality of life rather than curative interventions for concomitant conditions**. Families and healthcare providers make decisions about medical evaluations and interventions, with discussions about whether the person is evaluated in an ED or admitted to a hospital. Additional treatment issues that may arise during this stage are:

- Discontinuing memantine and cholinesterase inhibitors
- Discontinuing preventive medications (e.g., statins for cholesterol)
- Foregoing diagnostic procedures for nonacute symptoms
- Adhering to therapeutic diets
- Initiating a referral for hospice services
- Discontinuing or initiating dialysis or tube feeding

When these decisions are being discussed or becoming imminent, **nurses can suggest that a referral for hospice be considered**. It is not necessary to know for certain that the person meets specific criteria because a hospice nurse or social worker will assess the situation and meet with designated decision makers to discuss services, determine eligibility, and advise the family. Many hospice programs provide palliative care to address comfort and symptom management for patients with chronic declining conditions who are not ready for hospice.

Fast Facts

Nurses can encourage families and designated decision makers to initiate a phone call to hospice programs to find out about this resource for people with advanced dementia.

CULTURAL CONSIDERATIONS

Cultural factors can strongly influence many aspects of decision-making during advanced dementia. Examples of some differences regarding the meaning of continuing nutrition at the end of life are as follows (Marcolini, Putnam, & Aydin, 2018):

- In Western cultures, eating is paramount to survival, and lack of nutrition accelerates death.
- In Hindu tradition, decreasing oral intake at the end of life is viewed as a voluntary action done to prepare for a dignified death.

- The Taiwanese cultural belief is that a person should not die hungry because this would cause his or her soul to be restless.

Be open-minded and nonjudgmental about decisions related to artificial nutrition and hydration.

NURSING CARE FOR COMFORT

People with advanced dementia need physical and emotional comfort, but they are unable to verbally express these needs. Interventions that nurses can incorporate in usual care activities include the following:

- Assume that the person understands the meaning of nonverbal communication and is aware of what you are communicating with body language.
- Avoid being abrupt or hurried in verbal and nonverbal interactions.
- Make a warm and personal connection with the person by smiling, touching gently, using a soft voice, and making eye contact.
- Avoid disrespectful terminology.
- Anticipate needs related to pain, discomfort, positioning, food, fluids, toileting, and level of physical activity.
- Provide a therapeutic environment by controlling noise and lighting as much as possible (e.g., turn televisions to soothing music rather than to verbally intense programs).

Fast Facts

Assume that people with advanced dementia understand verbal and nonverbal communication and communicate in a respectful and caring manner at all times.

References

Marcolini, E. G., Putnam, A. T., & Aydin, A. (2018). History and perspectives on nutrition and hydration at the end of life. *Yale Journal of Biology and Medicine, 91*, 173–176.

McInerney, F., Doherty, K., Bindoff, A., Robinson, A., & Vickers, J. (2018). How is palliative care understood in the context of dementia? Results from a massive open online course. *Palliative Medicine, 32*(3), 594–602. doi:10.1177/0269216317743433

Van Wijngaarden, E., Alma, M., & The, A-M. (2019). "The eyes of others" are what really matters: The experience of living with dementia from an insider perspective. *PLoS One, 14*(4), e0214724. doi:10.1371/journal.pone.0214724

RESOURCES

National Hospice and Palliative Care Organization

https://www.nhpco.org

- Information about hospice and palliative care for people with dementia

National Institute on Aging

https://www.nia.nih.gov/health/end-life-care-people-dementia

- Information about end-of-life care in people with dementia

IV

Nursing Strategies to Address Emotional Needs and Behavioral Issues

10

Emotional Needs of People With Dementia and Their Care Partners

INTRODUCTION

People with dementia and all those in close relationships with them experience a "roller coaster" of many emotions beginning during the prediagnostic stage and usually continuing for years. This chapter discusses some of the most commonly experienced emotional responses and provides guidelines for nursing interventions to support people with dementia and their families.

In this chapter, you will learn:

1. Emotional needs of people with dementia and their families
2. Emotional needs during stages of dementia
3. Depression and antidepressants
4. Emotional needs of caregivers

EMOTIONAL NEEDS OF PEOPLE WITH DEMENTIA AND THEIR FAMILIES

Even for the most well-adjusted person, the diagnosis of dementia is a life-altering event with major implications, not only for the person with dementia but also for those close to that person. Even during the prediagnosis stage, the changes in memory, cognition, personality, behaviors, and level of independent functioning present emotional challenges to the person who experiences them and to all those in close contact with that person. Because the symptoms typically occur gradually and intermittently over a period of years, all those involved experience chronic uncertainty and a constant roller-coaster experience of emotional responses. As summarized by one person with dementia, "your life's torn and you need to abide by a whole new set of rules" (Sharp, 2019, p. 1435). An almost universal theme that begins at diagnosis and continues throughout the condition is the uncertainty of the progression and worries about the future.

In the words of a family member of a person with dementia:

One of the things I hate about Alzheimer's progression is the uncertainty to it all. . . . In most other illnesses there is a path that is followed. In normal situations you can apply logic and be fairly certain of an outcome. With Alzheimer's there is no logic; there is no normal. (Kannaley, Mehta, Yelton, & Friedman, 2019, p. 8)

Fast Facts

Be aware of the emotional challenges associated with the uncertainty about the effects of dementia on all those affected.

EMOTIONAL NEEDS DURING STAGES OF DEMENTIA

Emotional responses during the onset of manifestations and early diagnosis typically include loss, fear, worry, sadness, anxiety, denial, and withdrawal from usual activities. In recent years, people with early-stage dementia have shared their experiences through books, films, blogs, interviews, and other publicly available media, and healthcare professionals and Alzheimer's advocacy groups have published references and reports on the expressed needs of people with early-stage dementia. **An overriding theme expressed by people with early-stage dementia is that myths and misconceptions lead to stigma and misunderstanding**, which affect their relationships with family, friends, colleagues, and healthcare professionals.

In the words of three people recently diagnosed with Alzheimer's disease:

> We are happy with the support we have from all sides now. Really . . . really . . . But I still feel hopeless. Presumably you can hear it in the tone of my voice, both helpless and hopeless. (van Wijngaarden, Alma, & The, 2019, p. 12)

> I just hide from everybody. . . . I'll go in the bathroom and cry, and try to let it out, then tension out. (Portacolone, Johnson, Covinsky, Halpern, & Rubinstein, 2018, p. 11)

> After receiving the diagnosis, I was constantly thinking of it. In fact, I often lay awake all night, which was really an attack on my body, but even more on my mind. You know, if I cannot sleep, lots of things go through my mind. It's one large teeming snake pit then, this head of mine, a teeming snake pit. At that moment nothing is good, everything is negative. (van Wijngaarden et al., 2019, p. 8)

Emotional needs of people with dementia and their caregivers that are pertinent to nurses providing person-centered care include:

- Talking about their condition but not being stereotyped
- Having people listen to and treat them as individuals
- Expressing feelings about the effects of their condition
- Having people recognize and respect both their abilities and limitations
- Being asked about how they cope with the challenges of their condition
- Receiving support from professionals about their positive coping mechanisms
- Maintaining independent functioning in daily activities
- Talking about the ways in which others can be helpful
- Participating in support and educational groups
- Maintaining continuity with past interests, relationships, and social roles
- Developing new interests that are consistent with current abilities
- Connecting with others who have dementia or are caregivers
- Finding reliable information and resources

As dementia progresses to the moderate and later stages, people with dementia will have increasing difficulty expressing their

needs verbally. As discussed in Chapter 11, Dementia-Associated Behaviors, it is imperative to recognize behavioral and psychological symptoms of dementia that may be expressions of unmet emotional needs. A "rule of thumb" to keep in mind, especially when the person with dementia cannot express feelings verbally, is that **any behaviors should be responded to by addressing underlying emotional needs.** Even the most nonverbal person may be expressing emotional needs. It is important that even when a person with dementia cannot directly express emotional needs, he or she is able to receive emotional support from caregivers.

Fast Facts

People with dementia often express emotional needs behaviorally rather than verbally.

DEPRESSION

Depression is the most common psychological symptom in dementia, occurring in about half of the people with dementia. Characteristics of depression in people with dementia differ from those in people without dementia in the following ways: higher prevalence of symptoms related to motivation, fatigue, apathy, and psychomotor function and lower prevalence of anxiety, depressed mood, low self-esteem, and feelings of guilt. Caregivers of people with dementia are also at high risk for depression. Screen for depression in older adults who can communicate verbally by asking the following two questions:

- During the past 2 weeks, have you had little interest or pleasure in doing things?
- During the past 2 weeks (or month), have you often felt down, depressed, or hopeless?

Each question is scored as follows: not at all = 0, several days = 1, more than half of the days = 2, and nearly all the days = 3. A total score of 3 indicates the need for further evaluation.

Cultural Considerations

Cultural factors can influence the manifestations of depression, for example, through bodily symptoms, such as pain or headache. Also, in some cultural groups, feelings of depression may be considered shameful. Nurses can ask about feelings of "sadness" rather than depression.

Antidepressants

Much evidence supports the use of antidepressants for people with both dementia and depression; however, these drugs are also associated with significant adverse effects. Selective serotonin reuptake inhibitors (SSRIs) are the type of antidepressant most commonly used for people with dementia.

Examples of SSRIs are:

- Citalopram (Celexa)
- Escitalopram (Lexapro)
- Fluvoxamine (Luvox)
- Paroxetine (Paxil)
- Sertraline (Zoloft)

Consider all the following principles related to antidepressants for people with dementia:

- Antidepressants are appropriate, and often underutilized, for treatment of depression in people with dementia.
- Antidepressants may alleviate behaviors that are due to depression, such as emotional lability, decreased concentration, sleep disturbances, and diminished appetite.
- Immediate improvement will not be evident, but the medication should be given a fair trial (i.e., as long as 12 weeks) as long as serious adverse effects do not occur.
- Common adverse effects of antidepressants include nausea, vomiting, diarrhea, headache, nervousness, insomnia, tremor, dry mouth, and sexual dysfunction.
- Antidepressants cannot be used on an "as needed" (PRN) basis.

EMOTIONAL NEEDS OF CAREGIVERS

Family members and friends of people with dementia experience many of the same emotions as the person with dementia, frequently requiring shifts in emotions and coping during years of transitions between stages and uncertainty about what comes next. A major challenge, particularly for spouses and adult children who assume primary caregiving roles, is adjusting to major relationship changes and establishing "normalcy." Studies emphasize that striving to construct and sustain normalcy helps caregivers (especially spouses) focus on maintaining the "personhood" of both the person with dementia and the caregiver (Hale et al., 2019).

Nurses who care for people with dementia are frequently aware of caregiver needs, which are likely to be exacerbated during times of hospitalization and other medical instabilities. The term **caregiver burden** describes the emotional, physical, social, financial, and spiritual negative effects experienced by those who have caregiver responsibility for a family member with dementia.

Manifestations of Caregiver Burden

- Depression
- Disturbed sleep
- Social isolation
- Job interruption
- Financial difficulties
- Lack of time for self
- Poor physical health
- Psychological, emotional, and mental strain
- Feelings of anger, guilt, grief, anxiety, hopelessness, and helplessness

In the words of a spouse of a person with dementia:

> There are times when his lack of memory and thinking ability get to me. I have to put a positive attitude on, so I can cope with the daily actions that remind me of a dismal future. (Herron, Funk, & Spencer, 2019, p. e473)

In contrast to the emphasis on caregiver burden, gerontologists and geriatric practitioners have increasingly focused on identifying both the benefits and burdens of caregiving. In reality, most caregivers experience a combination of stresses and satisfactions. **Positive aspects of caregiving** include the following:

- A sense of accomplishment and gratification
- A sense of personal growth and purpose in life
- Experience of social approval
- Increased patience and acceptance
- Finding meaning in a new role

Cultural Considerations

Studies have found that minority older adults with dementia tended to be diagnosed later and have delayed help-seeking (Cheng, Au, Losada, Thompson, & Gallagher-Thompson, 2019). Nurses can suggest culturally appropriate community resources, such as those that may be available through local cultural groups for older adults.

Roles of Nurses Related to Caregivers' Emotional Needs

Nurses caring for people with dementia in short-term settings cannot address all the identified needs of caregivers; however, be aware of the manifestations of caregiver burden and express compassion. In addition, teach about the resources discussed in this chapter and encourage caregivers to participate in support and educational groups that address their concerns. Nurses also have essential roles in teaching caregivers about techniques to manage care issues, as discussed in Chapter 11, Dementia-Associated Behaviors, Chapter 12, Roles of Nurses in Specific Care Settings, Chapter 13, Issues Related to Daily Activities, Chapter 14, Addressing Safety Issues: Falls, Restraints, Wandering, and Chapter 15, Nursing Assessment and Management of Pain in People With Dementia. Moreover, nurses can support caregiver wellness through statements such as "It must be a challenge to care for _____, what do you do for your own wellness?"

Fast Facts

Address caregiver needs by teaching and demonstrating methods for managing care and suggesting resources for information and support.

References

Cheng, S. T., Au, A., Losada, A., Thompson, L. W., & Gallagher-Thompson, D. (2019). Psychological interventions for dementia caregivers: What we have achieved, what we have learned. *Current Psychiatry Reports, 21*(7), 59. doi:10.1007/s11920-019-1045-9

Hale, L., Mayland, E., Jenkins, M., Buttery, Y., Norris, P., Butler, M., & Kayes, N. (2019). Constructing normalcy in dementia care: Carers' perceptions of their roles and the supports they need. *The Gerontologist*. doi:10.1093/geront/gnz151

Herron, R., Funk, L., & Spencer, D. (2019). Responding the "Wrong way": The emotional work of caring for a family member with dementia. *The Gerontologist, 59*(5), e470–e478. doi:10.1093/geront/gnz047

Kannaley, K., Mehta, S., Yelton, B., & Friedman, D. B. (2019). Thematic analysis of blog narratives written by people with Alzheimer's disease and other dementias and care partners. *Dementia, 18*(7–8), 3071–3090. doi:10.1177/1471301218768162.

Portacolone, E., Johnson, J. K., Covinsky, K. E., Halpern, J., & Rubinstein, R. L. (2018). The effects and meanings of receiving a diagnosis of mild cognitive impairment or Alzheimer's disease when one lives alone. *Journal of Alzheimer's Disease, 61*(4), 1517–1529. doi:10.3233/JAD-170723

Sharp, B. K. (2019). Stress as experienced by people with dementia: An interpretive phenomenological analysis. *Dementia, 18*(4), 1427–1445. doi:10.1177/1471301217713877

Van Wijngaarden, E., Alma, M., & The, A-M. (2019). "The eyes of others" are what really matters: The experience of living with dementia from an insider perspective. *PLoS One, 14*(4), e0214724. doi:10.1371/journal.pone.0214724

11

Dementia-Associated Behaviors

INTRODUCTION

The term dementia-associated behavior *refers to commonly occurring behavioral problems that develop in addition to cognitive impairment in people with dementia. Although irreversible brain changes are the underlying cause, these behaviors often are precipitated by conditions that can be controlled. In some instances, interventions can prevent these behaviors. In all instances, nurses assess the person with dementia and implement appropriate interventions to address these challenging behaviors. This chapter presents an overview of common misunderstandings about dementia-associated behaviors and provides a more in-depth discussion of several types of behaviors that nurses address in clinical settings.*

In this chapter, you will learn:

1. Misunderstandings about dementia-associated behaviors
2. Behavioral and psychological symptoms of dementia (BPSD)
3. Nursing assessment of BPSD
4. Nursing interventions for BPSD
5. Pharmacological interventions

MISUNDERSTANDINGS ABOUT DEMENTIA-ASSOCIATED BEHAVIORS

An accurate interpretation of dementia-associated behaviors is based on knowledge not only about the person with dementia but also about potential contributing conditions. Dementia-associated behaviors are often misunderstood for reasons such as the following:

- Generalizations about people with dementia, such as "People with dementia become violent"
- Difficulty distinguishing between usual personality patterns and behaviors arising from dementia
- Inaccurately attributing behaviors to intentional actions
- Frequent or periodic fluctuations in behaviors, which makes it all the more difficult to assess or understand

Table 11.1 lists some common misunderstandings about behaviors and possible underlying causes. Nurses can use this information as a

Table 11.1

Misunderstandings and Possible Explanations Related to Dementia-Associated Behaviors

Misunderstandings	Possible Explanations
"He refuses to . . ."	He is unable to understand the command or carry out the required action; wants to do something else before agreeing to the activity; or wants to participate in the decision.
"She fights me when I . . ."	She may be experiencing pain or discomfort, which is exacerbated by the activity; she feels threatened by the actions.
Challenging or disruptive behavior	The behavior is a way to express a need or cope with stressful situations.
"He denies any problem."	He may not have insight, awareness, or ability to understand.
"There's no reason for him to act that way."	There usually is a triggering event or an unmet need.
Manipulative, deliberate actions to get attention	The person may not have enough insight or intent to be manipulative; the actions may be the only way the person is able to express needs.
Thinking that interventions that were effective in the past will continue to be effective	If the usual interventions no longer work, be flexible, creative, and try something else; use a "trial and error" approach by trying variations of interventions that worked.

guide to gaining an understanding of the meaning behind a patient's behaviors

Teach families about the realities of dementia-associated behaviors and avoid terminology or actions that perpetuate misunderstandings. For example, avoid saying "He refuses . . ." when the person with dementia is unable to understand the request.

Cultural Considerations

The cultural background of family caregivers may influence their perceptions of dementia-associated behaviors. Some beliefs and perceptions may be based on their experiences or hearsay about relatives who were labeled as "senile" decades ago. Nurses have important roles in providing accurate information about dementia-associated behaviors and appropriate ways to prevent and manage these behaviors.

BEHAVIORAL AND PSYCHOLOGICAL SYMPTOMS OF DEMENTIA

BPSD is the term used internationally to describe signs and symptoms that co-occur with cognitive symptoms in nearly all people with dementia during the illness course (Kales, Gitlin, & Lyketos, 2019). This term includes all the following behaviors:

- Mood disturbances: apathy, depression, euphoria, emotional lability
- Psychotic symptoms: delusions, hallucinations
- Agitation (verbal, vocal, or physical)
- Anxiety
- Personality changes
- Disinhibition
- Aberrant motor movements: pacing, wandering, rummaging
- Changes in sleep, eating, appetite

People with dementia are likely to manifest one or several BPSD during different stages, with symptoms developing and resolving intermittently and often concurrently. It is beyond the scope of this chapter to address all types of BPSD, but information in many other chapters of this text applies to this topic. This chapter addresses altered perception of reality and aggressive behaviors as two types of BPSD that nurses commonly address across clinical settings.

Altered Perception of Reality

People with dementia, especially during moderate and later stages, likely experience an altered perception of reality in many ways. The phrase altered perception of reality refers to **a continuum of symptoms, ranging from relatively simple misperceptions and illusions to more persistent hallucinations or delusions**. Visual and auditory hallucinations occur in people with dementia, particularly during moderate and advanced stages. Vivid or complex visual hallucinations are particularly common with Lewy body dementia and may develop earlier than in other types of dementia. Common themes of dementia-associated delusions include people stealing their belongings, feeling lost or abandoned, or spousal infidelity. These delusions are due to pathological changes of dementia and should not be labeled as paranoia or suspiciousness.

Effects of these misperceptions also vary, ranging from annoyances for others to severe anxiety and risks to safety for the person with dementia. In most situations, misperceptions do not need to be corrected, and usually the best intervention is to overlook them or provide accurate information in a matter-of-fact manner. Even when misperceptions are harmless, however, assess and document these as indicators of mental status. Interventions need to be initiated under the following circumstances:

- The misperceptions indicate a change in mental status that requires further assessment.
- The misperceptions cause distress or anxiety for the person with dementia or others.
- The person with dementia or others are going to take inappropriate action based on the misperception.
- The misperception poses a risk to the person with dementia or others.

⟳ Clinical Snapshot

Mr. C's son has assumed all responsibility for financial management because his father is no longer able to write checks or keep track of his bank accounts. Mr. C tells you that his son has stolen all his money and spends it on "drinking and carousing."

Distraction, or redirection of attention, is often an effective intervention, especially when you can get the person to focus on pleasant, comforting, or health-promoting activities (e.g., music, food, walking, or conversing about happy memories). Provision of reality-based information is sometimes helpful and therapeutic; however, in some circumstances, this action may increase the person's distress. For example, people with dementia may forget that a spouse or parent is deceased, and they may repeatedly inquire about that person. The traditional reality orientation approach would be to remind them the person is dead, but this may not be the most therapeutic response. In these situations, reminders that the person is dead often precipitate new or renewed feelings of grief and many questions about why the person with dementia was not told before. Nursing actions to address these kinds of situations include the following:

- Avoid discussion of details but address feelings ("You must miss your mother a lot. Are you feeling sad right now?").
- Distract with questions or activities ("I'm sorry your husband can't be here now. Tell me about your wedding").
- Communicate a sense of safety ("Your mother isn't here, but she is fine").
- If the person starts to cry and express sadness or grief, offer support but do not discourage expression of feelings unless the emotions are too distressful or prolonged.
- Use nonverbal communication to promote a sense of calm and caring.

Fast Facts

Identifying the most therapeutic response to address misperceptions of reality is often a "trial and error" process. Nurses can ask families and care partners about interventions that have worked for them and incorporate these into the care plan.

Aggressive Behaviors

People with dementia may exhibit aggressive behaviors such as hitting, biting, slapping, scratching, punching, grabbing, and kicking. **Nurses are most likely to encounter these behaviors when they are in close proximity to people with dementia during care activities.** Aggressive behaviors usually arise out of confusion as an act of protection from perceived harm or threat. Aggressive behaviors also arise because people with dementia feel little or no control over actions being imposed on them by others. Nursing interventions focus on preventing aggressive behaviors, de-escalating the behaviors, and protecting all people involved, as described in Exhibit 11.1.

Exhibit 11.1

Nursing Actions to Address Aggressive Behaviors

Nursing Actions to Prevent Aggressive Behaviors

- Identify conditions, including personal care activities, that are likely to precipitate aggressive behaviors.
- Incorporate information in care plans about effective ways of preventing aggressive behaviors.
- Use a calm and unhurried approach when initiating care activities.
- Avoid conditions that increase anxiety: noise, overstimulating environment, more than one staff approaching or talking with the person.
- Observe for indicators of behaviors escalating toward aggression (e.g., muscle tension, raising arms, facial expressions, and vocalizations) and initiate interventions.

Nursing Actions When Aggressive Behaviors Are Observed

- Step out of the reach of the person with dementia as soon as you observe indicators of potential aggressive acts.
- Use a calm and reassuring voice and demeanor.
- If you feel anxious or are hurried, take time to become centered and calm before and during interactions and patient care activities.
- Clearly and simply describe each step related to care activities before and during your nursing actions.
- When aggression is a reaction to the person's loss of control over his or her care, incorporate interventions that address autonomy and perceived control (e.g., facilitating as much independence as possible, even when it is more time-consuming; asking "Is it okay if I . . . ?").
- Use a gentle touch, while also providing appropriate personal space.
- Address the feelings of the person with dementia ("This may seem frightening to you, but you are safe, and we are helping you to be comfortable in bed").
- Keep the person's close environment clear of objects that can be thrown, broken, or cause harm.

Actions to Take if the Aggressive Behaviors Are Potentially Harmful

- Use nonthreatening actions for self-protection: Use your free hand to pry fingers away when someone grabs your arm.
- Protect yourself by keeping at arm's length or being out of reach as much as possible.
- Tell the person that the behavior is unacceptable by using a simple statement ("That hurts. Stop kicking").

- When absolutely necessary, use a method of holding the patient to prevent harm; move the person into a safe position as soon as possible.
- Once the person with dementia is in a safe position, have only one staff interact if this is safe for all involved.

When precipitating conditions cannot be identified or when aggressive behaviors occur frequently and do not seem to be related to care activities, an interdisciplinary team of healthcare professionals needs to address the behaviors. For example, because aggressive behaviors can be a symptom of delirium, nurses need to consider all causative conditions discussed in Chapter 2, Conditions That Affect Cognitive Function. Aggressive behaviors may also be caused by pain or discomfort, even when the person does not appear to be in pain, as discussed in Chapter 15, Nursing Assessment and Management of Pain in People With Dementia.

Fast Facts

When people with dementia exhibit aggressive behaviors, nurses need to provide for the safety of the person with dementia and others who are involved.

NURSING ASSESSMENT OF BPSD

Nurses are responsible for identifying precipitating conditions of BPSD as well as the actual and potential detrimental effects of the behaviors. For example, it is imperative to assess whether the effects are annoying, stressful, risky, or seriously unsafe for the person with dementia or for any of those around the person. This is an important aspect of assessment because nurses need to immediately address behaviors that are unsafe or arise out of unmet needs. On the other hand, it may be appropriate to ignore, tolerate, or even support behaviors that do not affect safety, comfort, or quality of life. In all situations, an accurate assessment of both causes and effects is essential for planning appropriate nursing actions. Nurses can use the following kinds of questions to assess BPSD:

- Is the person expressing a physical need?
- Is the person expressing an emotional need?

- Do the behaviors arise primarily out of confusion, lack of awareness, or misperceptions?
- Do the behaviors pose risks or are they unsafe for the person with dementia?
- Are the behaviors distressing or bothersome for the person with dementia?
- Do the behaviors pose risks for people around the person with dementia (e.g., family, care partners, healthcare providers, or others in the immediate environment)?
- Are the behaviors annoying or bothersome to other people but not to the person with dementia?

Fast Facts

Assess both the causes and the effects of BPSD and plan nursing interventions accordingly. BPSD may be an important indicator of a change in mental status, which can be due to any of the conditions discussed in Chapter 2, Conditions That Affect Cognitive Function.

🔵 Clinical Snapshot

Nurses know that Mrs. N loudly calls "Sink, sink, I'm sinking" when she needs to void, and they assist her immediately because otherwise she will attempt to get out of bed by herself and she is unsteady. As the nurse is assisting, Mrs. N says, "My mother usually helps me, but she's at the store now." The nurse responds, "I'm glad I can be here to help."

NURSING INTERVENTIONS FOR BPSD

Management of BPSD requires a multifaceted approach that is based on a comprehensive care plan developed with input from families, care partners, and interprofessional healthcare providers. When family caregivers have been caring for the person with dementia, first ask them about techniques to prevent and manage BPSD. Nonpharmacological approaches are considered the first line of management before initiating medications, which are discussed in the next section. Recent reviews of research identify the following types of interventions as the most effective for BPSD:

- Identification and management of contributing causes, such as interventions for pain

- Person-centered approaches, including meaningful activities
- Reminiscence therapy
- Sensory-focused interventions, such as massage, music therapy, and aromatherapy
- Pet therapy with dogs or stuffed or robotic pets
- Education of all caregivers (Kales, Lyketsos, Miller, & Ballard, 2019; Legere, McNeill, Schendel Martin, Acorn, & An, 2018; Scales, Zimmerman, & Miller, 2018; Smith & D'Amico, 2019)

Modifying the personal environment is another intervention because dementia impairs one's ability to interpret and respond to environmental stimuli. Although nurses have limited control over patients' environments, some relatively simple actions they can take when caring for people with dementia include:

- Adjusting room temperature for the person's comfort
- Providing blankets (even warmed ones) when patients are cold
- Adjusting lighting in the room
- Adjusting television to appropriate channels or keeping it off
- Providing favorite music
- Promoting a "culture of quiet and calm" in and around patient rooms
- Suggesting that family bring in photos and other reminders of loved ones

In the words of a nursing assistant:

> I think it's too many people, too big a place and I think that gets her a bit more agitated. . . . Even when you try and give her something else to do it doesn't last for very long. . . . We have tried so very many things. (Watson, 2019, p. 557)

PHARMACOLOGICAL INTERVENTIONS

The use of antipsychotic agents to treat BPSD was common until the early 2000s, when gerontological professionals raised concerns about serious adverse effects and lack of efficacy, based on a wide base of research. By 2008, the Food and Drug Administration (FDA) had issued "black box warnings" advising against the use of antipsychotic agents for BPSD. In 2012, the Centers for Medicare and Medicaid Services launched the National Partnership to Improve Dementia Care in Nursing Homes, and many national organizations of gerontological healthcare professionals issued mandates and guidelines aimed at reducing the use of antipsychotics in people with dementia.

Evidence-Based Guidelines for BPSD

■ Psychotropic medications are a last resort for BPSD and should be initiated only after other measures have been tried and when the behaviors are unsafe or cause serious distress.
■ Use lowest effective dose and monitor for adverse effects.
■ Adverse effects of antipsychotics include restlessness, incontinence, stroke, dry mouth, constipation, cognitive decline, parkinsonism, diabetes, and depression.
■ Review all psychotropic medications at least once every 3 months and consider dose reduction or discontinuation.
■ Review all psychotropic medications whenever there is a change in the person's condition or environment (e.g., when admitted to the hospital and upon discharge).
■ Carefully weigh the risks versus benefits before initiating pharmacological interventions.

Fast Facts

Pharmacological interventions are used only as a last resort for BPSD because of their limited efficacy and high risk for adverse effects. When they are prescribed, they should be of the lowest dose for the shortest time, and nurses need to observe for adverse effects.

References

Kales, H. C., Gitlin, L. N., & Lyketsos, C. G. (2019). When less is more, but still not enough: Why focusing on limiting antipsychotics in people with dementia is the wrong policy imperative. *Journal of the American Medical Directors Association, 20,* 1074–1079. doi:10.1016/j.jamda.2019.05.022

Kales, H. C., Lyketsos, C. G., Miller, E. M., & Ballard, C. (2019). Management of behavioral and psychological symptoms in people with Alzheimer's disease: An international Delphi consensus. *International Psychogeriatrics, 31*(1), 83–90. doi:10.1017/S1041610218000534

Legere, L. E., McNeill, S., Schendel Martin, L., Acorn, M, & An, D. (2018). Nonpharmacological approaches for behavioural and psychological symptoms of dementia in older adults: A systematic review of reviews. *Journal of Clinical Nursing, 27*(7–8), e1360–e1376. doi:10.1111/jocn.14007

Scales, K., Zimmerman, S., & Miller, S. (2018). Evidence-based nonpharmacological practices to address behavioral and psychological symptoms of dementia. *The Gerontologist, 58*(S1), S88–S102. doi:10.1093/geront/gnx167

Smith, B. C., & D'Amico, M. (2019). Sensory-based interventions for adults with dementia and Alzheimer's disease: A scoping review. *Occupational Therapy and Health Care,* 1–31. doi:10.1080/07380577.2019.1608488

Watson, J. (2019). Developing the senses framework to support relationship-centred care for people with advanced dementia until the end of life in care homes. *Dementia, 18*(2), 545–566. doi:10.1177/1471301216682880

RESOURCES

Alzheimer's Association

https://www.alz.org

- Information for professionals and families about dementia-associated behaviors

Hartford Institute for Geriatric Nursing

https://consultgeri.org/try-this/dementia/issue-d4

- Information on how to develop therapeutic activity kits for people with dementia

V

Nursing Strategies to Address Issues Related to Care

12

Roles of Nurses in Specific Care Settings

INTRODUCTION

Nurses who care for older adults in any healthcare setting are likely to care for patients who have dementia as a secondary diagnosis. It is not unusual or unprofessional to feel frustrated and unprepared and view these situations as challenging and time-consuming. Because the primary focus in usual healthcare settings is on the presenting medical problems, issues related to dementia may be overlooked. In these situations, dementia can be viewed as a chronic condition that interacts with additional chronic medical conditions (a) to complicate the overall situation, (b) to be exacerbated during hospitalizations for medical or surgical events, (c) as requiring ongoing assessment, (d) as requiring additional interventions be incorporated into the usual care plan, and (e) as presenting unique challenges and opportunities for providing person-centered care. Although nurses generally have guidelines for managing chronic medical conditions, they are less likely to have clear guidelines related to the needs of people who have dementia. This chapter focuses on dementia-related issues that nurses commonly address when they work in specific healthcare settings.

In this chapter, you will learn:

1. Overview of challenges in caring for patients with dementia in acute care settings
2. Nursing strategies to obtain accurate information
3. Detecting elder abuse in acute care settings
4. Resources within hospitals
5. Considerations related to skilled care and rehabilitation settings

OVERVIEW

Older adults with dementia are more likely than those without this diagnosis to be admitted to a hospital or seen in an ED (Kent et al., 2019; Sommerlad et al., 2019). Studies indicate that people with dementia are at higher risk for serious consequences of hospitalization-associated delirium, iatrogenic complications, and cognitive and functional decline (Maust, Kim, Chiang, Langa, & Kales, 2019). Even though dementia is a common diagnosis, it will not necessarily be documented on the patient's chart if it is not the primary reason for the admission.

Because dementia develops gradually and can be exacerbated by a medical condition or disruption in the person's routine, the hospitalization itself may become the "straw that breaks the camel's back" that raises questions about dementia as a probable diagnosis. In these situations, address issues related to diagnosing the change in mental status. If you suspect that a patient has undiagnosed dementia, use the family questionnaire or patient behavior assessment tool listed in the Resources section at the end of this chapter. Information in this chapter is pertinent to caring for patients who have dementia in institutional settings, including EDs, acute care facilities, and rehabilitation settings.

OBTAINING ACCURATE INFORMATION

Nurses in EDs often care for patients with dementia who arrive for an evaluation of a change in mental status or for treatment of injuries sustained during a fall. Often, there is little or no reliable information about the person's usual level of functioning and baseline mental status. Accurate information about medications and medical diagnoses also may be lacking.

Another challenge is that patients with moderate dementia or expressive aphasia may report something different from the reported presenting problem. For example, they may not be able to verbally describe their symptoms or they may use words that do not accurately describe the location of pain. And when asked about pain or other symptoms, their "yes" or "no" answers may not be accurate. In addition, the person's mental status is likely to be compromised by the confusion of being in an unfamiliar environment. In these situations, it may be difficult to pinpoint the presenting problem.

In all these situations, obtain as much information as possible from the person with dementia and then confirm the accuracy of this information with someone who can verify or amplify the information. Some strategies for obtaining assessment information when caring for someone with dementia include:

- Check for any form of identification (i.e., medic alert bracelet, necklace, or wallet card) that includes a toll-free number to call for medical history and information about contact people. When you call the toll-free number, ask how recently this information was updated.
- Contact the person's care partners and request information.
- If the person came from a nursing facility, call and ask to talk with a staff member who is familiar with the patient and ask for baseline functioning and mental status, current medications, and for a detailed description of the reason for being sent for evaluation.
- Ask care partners to bring all containers from currently and recently used medications, including nonprescription products.
- Call the person's pharmacy to obtain information about current and recently prescribed medications.
- Review any electronic medical record available in your facility.

Fast Facts

Check for nonprescription medications that can affect mental status. For example, many people take diphenhydramine (Benadryl) as a sleep aid and do not recognize that this can cause cognitive impairment, especially in older adults.

Cultural Considerations

Patients with dementia with **limited English proficiency** (e.g., those whose primary language is not English) may have an additional barrier giving and receiving information. Nurses can request interpreter services that are available in all hospital settings. Although family may be able to interpret, professional interpreters are recommended for communication about medical issues.

MANAGING BEHAVIORAL MANIFESTATIONS

Another nursing challenge in acute care settings is addressing common behavioral manifestations, such as agitation and increased confusion. **These behaviors often pose safety issues**, such as falls, fall-related injuries, and dislodging of medically necessary equipment (e.g., oxygen cannulas and intravenous [IV] tubing). Hospitals often provide a bedside sitter service when patient behaviors are associated with safety concerns and no caregiver is available to accompany the patient. Nurses can anticipate the need for a bedside sitter and suggest the referral according to the hospital policy.

Another common issue for nurses in acute care settings is managing daily care activities for patients with dementia. In addition to the interventions discussed in Chapters 11 through 15 in this book, it is important to obtain information about effective interventions that were used by care partners before the patient was hospitalized. This information can be gathered by talking with the patient's care partners when they visit and by calling nursing staff or family members who provided care in the home or long-term care settings. Incorporate this information into the care plan and communicate pertinent and effective strategies during shift reports, especially for patients who cannot readily communicate about their needs.

DETECTING ELDER ABUSE

Be on the alert not only for obvious manifestations of elder abuse (e.g., bruises, suspicious injuries) but also for subtle signs of abuse or self-neglect (e.g., malnutrition and medication mismanagement).

Nursing considerations related to detection of elder abuse include the following:

- If there are questions about malnutrition, suggest that a serum albumin level be obtained.
- If the person with dementia is brought to an ED because he or she is lost and cannot find the way home, consider that this can be a form of elder neglect.
- Observe interactions between the patient and any caregivers who are with the person and be alert to signs of abusive relationships

(e.g., caregiver talking inappropriately to the person with dementia).

■ Whenever there is suspicion of elder abuse or neglect, nurses have an obligation to follow the hospital protocol with regard to reporting and follow-up, as described in Chapter 16, Self-Neglect and Elder Abuse of People With Dementia.

RESOURCES WITHIN HOSPITALS

In recent years, many hospitals have initiated programs to address the unique needs of patients with dementia. Be aware of any available resources within your institution. Two outstanding initiatives that are widely available in hospitals throughout the United States are **Acute Care for the Elderly (ACE) units** and the **Nurses Improving Care for Healthsystem Elders (NICHE) program** of the Hartford Institute for Geriatric Nursing.

■ ACE units are designated hospital units that provide a multidisciplinary approach to preventing and managing complex geriatric syndromes. This model includes the following key elements: patient-centered care, interprofessional team management, frequent reassessments, early discharge planning, and a specialized physical environment. Nurses who work in a hospital that has an ACE unit can request a consultation about care of patients with dementia, including consideration that the patient be transferred to that unit.

■ An integral component of NICHE is the Geriatric Resource Nurse, a specially trained nurse consultant and role model for addressing complex geriatric situations, such as patients with dementia. In 2020, more than 700 hospitals in the United States provided NICHE services. Nurses who work in a NICHE hospital can request advice from one of these nurses to assist with the development of appropriate care plans for patients with dementia.

Nurses who do not have access to specialized resources or programs can suggest referrals for assessment and interventions to appropriate professional colleagues, including:

■ Geriatric clinical nurse specialist or geriatric resource nurse for assistance and consultation related to care planning

■ Geropsychiatrist, neurologist, or geriatrician for evaluation of mental status and recommendations about management

■ Social worker for discussions with care partners and assistance with discharge planning

- Social worker for information about helpful community services, such as the Alzheimer's Association
- Speech therapist for cognitive therapies
- Occupational therapist for safety and independence in activities of daily living (including driving rehabilitation)
- Physical therapist for maintaining safe mobility and preventing falls and excess disability
- Speech therapist for assessment and recommendations related to chewing, swallowing, and safe eating
- Pastoral care for assistance with spiritual care

TRANSITIONS IN CARE

As soon as a patient with dementia is admitted to any short-term care facility (e.g., acute care, EDs, rehabilitation or skilled care facility), **initiate discharge planning.** At a minimum, prior to discharge, provide the following patient education information both verbally and in writing: diagnosis, medications, referrals, and all follow-up appointments. Even for people with early-stage dementia, assure at least one caregiver also receives this information and has an opportunity to ask questions. When patients are transferred within institutional settings or taken to another unit for tests, it is helpful to have a family member or familiar staff person accompany the patient and assure that appropriate information is communicated verbally to supplement the information in the chart and to provide continuity and comfort to the person with dementia.

CONSIDERATIONS RELATED TO SKILLED CARE AND REHABILITATION SETTINGS

Skilled nursing care is defined as **medically necessary services for people who require daily or intermittent care provided by a registered nurse in a Medicare-certified facility or by a Medicare-certified home care agency**. Because skilled nursing services are short term and based on strict criteria, people with dementia often become disqualified before they or their care partners think they are ready for discharge. In these situations, nurses providing skilled care services to dementia patients in home or institutional settings need to be proactive in planning for the next level of care. One approach is to initiate a timely referral for available medical social work services as part of skilled care. Many of the necessary services for people who no longer qualify for skilled care are not covered by health insurance. Some services, however, may be covered by long-term care insurance for the small percentage of people who have purchased those policies. A medical social worker can assist families with decisions about resources as well as financial support for needed services. Nurses also can suggest referrals for the types of services that are available to address needs of people with dementia and their care partners, as discussed in Chapter 16.

Fast Facts

Because skilled nursing services are short term and the needs of patients with dementia are complex, nurses need to be proactive in planning continuity of care.

Clinical Snapshot

Ms. B was admitted for skilled therapy after surgery for a total hip replacement. Her daughter assumed she would be in the facility for several weeks, but Ms. B qualifies for only 9 days of therapy because she has moderate dementia and has not been able to learn how to use her walker without assistance. You suggest that Ms. B's daughter begin exploring options for care at home and you ask the social worker to provide information.

References

Kent, T., Lesser, A., Israni, J., Hwang, U., Carpenter, C., & Ko, K. J. (2019). 30-day emergency department revisit rates among older adults with dementia. *Journal of the American Geriatrics Society, 67*(11), 2254–2259. doi:10.1111/jgs.16114

Maust, D., Kim, H., Chiang, C., Langa, K. M., & Kales, H. C. (2019). Predicting risk of potentially preventable hospitalization in older adults with dementia. *Journal of the American Geriatrics Society, 67*(10), 2077–2084. doi:10.1111/jgs.16030

Sommerlad, A., Perera, G., Mueller, C., Singh-Manoux, A., Lewis, G., Stewart, R., & Livingston, G. (2019). Hospitalisation of people with dementia: Evidence from English health records from 2008 to 2016. *European Journal of Epidemiology, 34*(6), 567–577. doi:10.1007/s10654-019-00481-x

RESOURCES

Alzheimer's Association

https://www.alz.org

- Information to assist care partners in preparing for hospitalization of a person with dementia

Hartford Institute for Geriatric Nursing

https://consultgerirn.org/resources

- Recognition of Dementia in Hospitalized Older Adults, *Try This*, Issue D5, and video demonstrating application of the assessment tool
- Working With Families of Hospitalized Older Adults With Dementia, *Try This*, Issue D10, and video demonstrating application of the assessment tool

https://nicheprogram.org

- Knowledge center with "Need to Knows" information about care of patients with dementia in hospital settings
- Caregiver tools about issues related to care of people with dementia

13

Issues Related to Daily Activities

INTRODUCTION

People with dementia have difficulty performing daily care activities, and they depend on others to assist with their care. People with mild and moderate dementia usually have a routine that enables them to maintain some independence. They may depend on a step-by-step process or the provision of cues and verbal prompts. Any change in their environment or caregiver situation can disrupt their routines and increase their dependency on others. Nurses need to identify ways to support the person's ability to perform daily activities as much as possible, even when this is more time-consuming than doing the activities for the person.

In this chapter, you will learn:

1. How to identify the level of assistance that is most appropriate for the person with dementia
2. Nursing interventions to address issues related to eating
3. Nursing interventions to address issues related to bathing, dressing, and personal care
4. How to promote bladder and bowel continence
5. Nursing interventions to facilitate administration of medications and treatments
6. Nursing interventions to promote sleep

PROVIDING THE APPROPRIATE LEVEL OF CARE

A review of person-centered care practices for supporting daily activities in people with dementia identified the following essential components:

- Address both cognitive and functional decline as well as remaining abilities.
- Show respect and allow for individualized abilities, likes, and dislikes.
- Provide the level of assistance to support independence.
- Attend to dignity during all daily activities (Prizer & Zimmerman, 2018).

To provide person-centered care during **activities of daily living (ADL)**, add another layer of assessment focusing on strengths and abilities so as to support the person's highest level of function. Although this may take more time than providing care directly, it is an essential aspect of person-centered care. This approach prevents **excess disability**, which refers to limitations that unnecessarily interfere with someone's level of functioning. People with dementia frequently experience excess disability because the people with whom they interact do not understand how to promote their highest level of functioning.

Fast Facts

Nurses provide person-centered care and prevent excess disability when they develop a care plan based on an assessment of the person's strengths and abilities.

ASSESSING COGNITIVE ABILITIES

A person's ability to perform daily activities is affected by physical and cognitive skills. Whereas physical skills may be easy to assess, it is more challenging to assess cognitive skills that affect performance of daily activities. Whenever feasible, facilitate a referral for an occupational therapist to assess abilities and develop care plans for people with dementia. Ask families and care partners about interventions that facilitate the person's performance of ADL. People with mild dementia may be able to describe actions that support their ability to perform ADL as independently as possible. The following skills are involved in performing ADL:

- Initiate a task.
- Understand directions.
- Perform steps in the correct order.
- Maintain attention.
- Complete an activity.
- Imitate actions of others.

Use information about these cognitive skills as a guide to developing care plans supporting the optimal level of independence for people with dementia. The next sections of this chapter provide guidelines for addressing the daily activities that are most pertinent to care of people with dementia. Interventions for safe mobility are discussed in Chapter 14, Addressing Safety Issues.

Fast Facts

Assess cognitive skills and plan interventions that support the person's optimal level of functioning in daily activities. Whenever feasible, facilitate a referral for an occupational therapist to assess and develop a care plan for people with dementia.

ADDRESSING ISSUES RELATED TO EATING

Problems with eating occur during all stages of dementia, as illustrated in the following examples:

- Forgetting to eat
- Loss of appetite (sometimes due to medications, medical condition, or depression)
- Inability to prepare foods and lack of appropriate assistance or prompts
- Loss of ability to recognize food as something pleasurable
- Not understanding the tasks involved (e.g., not taking lids off containers or not opening individual condiment packages)
- Being in an unfamiliar and confusing environment
- Inability to maintain attention
- Difficulty chewing due to dental problems or not having comfortable dentures
- Difficulty chewing and swallowing due to advanced dementia or other pathologic conditions

- Increased risk of aspiration due to difficulty chewing and swallowing

Managing eating behaviors is an essential aspect of providing adequate nutrition and hydration. These issues are especially complex in the advanced stage of dementia because they involve ethical decisions related to the use of tube feedings, as discussed in Chapter 17, Ethical and Legal Issues.

Ask families and care partners about interventions they find effective to promote nutrition for the person with dementia, such as providing favorite foods and serving at the preferred temperature. Nurses also can initiate referrals for registered dieticians for assessment and interventions related to nutritional needs (including weight loss). When chewing or swallowing issues interfere with nutrition or increase the risk for choking and aspiration pneumonia, initiate a referral for speech and language therapists. If patients have difficulty filling out menus or following the procedure for ordering food and beverages, provide or arrange for appropriate assistance.

Nursing interventions that may be appropriate for addressing eating problems in people with dementia include:

- Opening containers, removing lids, and setting up trays so that food items are easily accessible
- Describing food items that the person may not recognize
- Providing small frequent meals rather than large meals
- Offering nutritious snacks and beverages
- Cutting food into bite-size pieces before presenting it
- Sitting face-to-face and using a friendly approach when feeding
- Providing appropriate verbal and nonverbal cues
- Using cups rather than bowls for soups and thin foods
- Adapting the environment as much as possible to control noise, distractions, and overstimulation

In the words of a nursing assistant:

> You don't force somebody if they don't want to eat and they are making that clear to you . . . so that's tough from our point of view because you want them to get their nutrition. (Watson, 2019, p. 553)

Fast Facts

Nurses work closely with families, care partners, dieticians, and speech therapists to identify interventions that are most effective for addressing nutritional needs of people with dementia.

ADDRESSING ISSUES RELATED TO BATHING, DRESSING, AND PERSONAL CARE

When people with dementia are in their usual settings they may have a routine that enables them to get dressed and carry out personal care activities. If they cannot maintain this routine, for example in a hospital setting, they are likely to be confused and may become resistant or even combative. The following nursing interventions may be appropriate when providing personal care for people with dementia:

- Find out the person's usual routine and adhere to it as closely as possible (e.g., same time of day, preferred method, best approach).
- Keep the care as simple as possible.
- Assess for pain or discomfort as possible causes of resistance and initiate interventions for pain management (see Chapter 15, Nursing Assessment and Management of Pain in People With Dementia).
- Encourage family or care partners to provide assistance as they usually do.
- Provide for privacy and comfort (e.g., keep the person covered, close bed curtains, and make sure the environment is warm).
- Observe whether the person performs oral care and provide assistance or prompts as necessary.
- Describe your actions in simple terms if the person feels threatened or does not understand what you are doing.
- If the person is physically aggressive or resistive, stop the task and address the behaviors; resume the task only when the person is calm and cooperative.
- Provide prompts for, or appropriate assistance with, hair care and shaving.
- If resources are available, ask care partners if they want to arrange for barber or beautician services.

Fast Facts

People with mild and moderate dementia usually have a routine that enables them to perform personal care activities with prompts, setups, or minimal assistance.

⟳ Clinical Snapshot

The care plan for Mr. C includes the following intervention: After breakfast and before bed, supervise Mr. C's oral care by putting

(continued)

(*continued*)

toothpaste on his toothbrush, placing it on the sink near a cup of water, and verbally prompting him to brush his teeth.

INTERVENTIONS TO PROMOTE BOWEL AND BLADDER CONTINENCE

Nursing interventions to help maintain continence can be very challenging because people with dementia gradually lose control of bowel and bladder elimination. Assess the person's usual pattern of bowel and bladder elimination and identify conditions likely to cause incontinence, such as the following:

- Unfamiliar environments, difficulty finding toileting facilities
- Not receiving timely and appropriate assistance with toileting needs
- Urinary tract infection
- Medical conditions (e.g., urinary retention, prostatic hypertrophy)
- Adverse medication effects (e.g., diuretics, narcotics, anticholinergics)
- Incontinence briefs that interfere with the person's ability to use a commode
- Functional limitations that affect the person's ability to get to a toilet in a timely manner

Even if dementia does not affect one's control over bowel and bladder elimination, it can affect one's ability to remember to use the toilet. Dementia also affects one's ability to report about bowel movements. Use any of the following strategies to promote continence in people with dementia:

- Observe patterns of bowel and bladder elimination; do not rely on the person to accurately self-report.
- Observe for and respond to signs that the person needs assistance with toileting.
- Develop a care plan for anticipating and addressing toileting needs (usually at 2-hour intervals during the day).
- Document frequency, amount, and consistency of bowel movements and be on the alert for signs of constipation.
- Provide cues and assistance at appropriate intervals.
- Make sure the bathroom is clearly marked and the pathway to it is uncluttered.
- Arrange for medical evaluation for conditions that may contribute to incontinence (e.g., urinary tract infection, enlarged prostate, urinary retention).
- If incontinence occurs, preserve the person's dignity and avoid any responses that may seem judgmental or patronizing.

- Provide assistance with or reminders about hand washing after using the bathroom.

Identify factors that affect bowel and bladder continence for each patient with dementia and plan individualized interventions to prevent episodes of incontinence.

⟳ **Clinical Snapshot**

Mrs. G's care plan includes the following: Patient becomes agitated if incontinence briefs are used; provide verbal prompts and stand-by assistance with walking to the bathroom every 3 hours during the day and once during the night when she is awake; observe toilet for stool and record in chart.

ADDRESSING ISSUES RELATED TO MEDICATIONS AND TREATMENTS

When nurses administer medications, take vital signs, or perform other direct care activities for patients who have dementia, they often deal with challenges such as:

- Refusal to take medications
- Difficulty swallowing medications
- Diminished ability or inability to understand directions or explanations
- Perception of threat in relation to invasive procedures (i.e., blood draws, injections)
- Fear of or experience of pain or discomfort due to being moved or repositioned
- Misperceptions of medical equipment

When people with dementia are resistant, or even combative, address conditions contributing to fear and misperceptions as discussed in Chapter 11, Dementia-Associated Behaviors. Additional interventions to facilitate direct care include the following:

- Ask families and care partners about their usual approaches.
- Offer medications with a simple statement, such as "It's time for you to have these." Use verbal and nonverbal prompts as appropriate.
- Unless contraindicated (e.g., enteric-coated or extended release), crush medications and mix with small amount of soft food that the person likes.

- If the person resists or has difficulty swallowing pills, consult with pharmacist about other forms of medications that are available and more acceptable (e.g., liquid, dissolving tablets, or patches).
- Do not argue with the person but use a direct and reassuring approach.
- Address pain and comfort conditions that may be causing resistance or refusal.
- If the person pulls at tubes, cover the tubing with loose fluffy bandages.
- Obtain assistance from family or staff to distract the person's attention while you are checking vital signs or performing nursing procedures.
- If the person is resistive or agitated, perform the care task at another time.
- If feasible, perform nursing procedures at the time of day when the person is usually more cooperative.

Fast Facts

Creative strategies are often needed for administering medications and treatments to people with dementia.

Clinical Snapshot

Mrs. G's daughter reports that her mother takes her pills if you crush them, put them in vanilla pudding, provide a cup of warm water, and say, "This is the pudding that Molly made for you and it has your pills in it to make you feel better."

NURSING INTERVENTIONS TO PROMOTE SLEEP

At least half of the people with dementia experience significant sleep disturbances, such as:

- Day–night sleep pattern reversal
- Frequent nighttime awakenings
- Fragmented sleep patterns
- Excessive daytime sleepiness
- Increased somnolence (15 or more hours/day, especially in very advanced dementia)

Typically a very early sign of Lewy body dementia, sleep disturbances are characterized by excessive daytime sleepiness and very active dreaming during sleep, sometimes accompanied by agitation. In all types of dementia, sleep disturbances are caused by pathological brain changes and can be exacerbated by coexisting conditions.

Coexisting Conditions Exacerbating Sleep Disturbances

- Pain
- Anxiety
- Delirium
- Depression
- Sleep apnea
- Medical conditions
- Restless legs syndrome
- Adverse medication effects

As with all conditions in people with dementia, identify factors contributing to sleep disturbances rather than attribute the problem solely to dementia. Assess and address pain in people with dementia, as discussed in Chapter 15, Nursing Assessment and Management of Pain in People With Dementia. Ask someone to stay with the person to provide comfort and reassurance until the person falls asleep. Talk with primary care practitioners to address medical conditions or adverse medication effects that can cause sleep disturbances.

If pharmacological interventions are necessary, be aware of the increased risk of serious adverse effects in older adults with dementia. Nonbenzodiazepine hypnotics used short-term for insomnia include:

- Eszopiclone (Lunesta)
- Ramelteon (Rozerem)
- Zaleplon (Sonata)
- Zolpidem (Ambien)

Sleep disorders due to Lewy body dementia need to be addressed by neurologists because of the unique characteristics of this type of dementia including their atypical reactions to medications.

Nurses can teach about nonpharmacological interventions that promote sleep such as the following:

- Try to maintain a regular daily schedule for sleep, rest, activity, and meals.
- Take a warm, relaxing bath in the afternoon or early evening.
- Encourage regular daily exercise and interesting physical activities.
- Address pain, anxiety, distress, and any other sources of discomfort.
- Encourage exposure to sunlight or full-spectrum lighting during the day.
- After 1 p.m., avoid foods, beverages, and medications that contain caffeine or stimulants (e.g., tea, cocoa, coffee, chocolate, sugar, refined carbohydrates, and some over-the-counter pain relievers and cold preparations).

- In the evening, drink beverages and eat snacks that promote sleep (e.g., warm milk, chamomile tea, and snacks with whole grains).
- Listen to soothing music.
- Make sure the bedroom temperature is comfortable.
- Control lighting and noise for optimal sleep conditions.
- In the evening and if the person wakens during the night, avoid activities that are stimulating or confusing (e.g., television, distracting conversations).
- Use lavender essential oil for aromatherapy.
- Use one or more of the following relaxation methods: imagery, meditation, deep breathing, progressive relaxation, body or foot massage, or rocking in a chair.

Fast Facts

Developing and incorporating relatively simple interventions known to be effective from family or caregivers can be useful in promoting sleep.

Clinical Snapshot

When Mr. N's son visits him in the evening, nurses bring chamomile tea from the beverage cart so that the son can encourage him to drink it.

References

Prizer, L., & Zimmerman, S. (2018). Progressive support for activities of daily living for persons living with dementia. *The Gerontologist, 58*(S1), S74–S87. doi:10.1093/geront/gnx103

Watson, J. (2019). Developing the Senses Framework to support relationship-centred care for people with advanced dementia until the end of life in care homes. *Dementia, 18*(2), 545–566. doi:10.1177/1471301216682880

RESOURCES

https://consultgeri.org

- Try This Series
- Eating and feeding issues in older adults with dementia: Assessment
- Eating and feeding issues in older adults with dementia: Interventions
- Oral healthcare
- Hydration management
- Sleep problems

14

Addressing Safety Issues: Falls, Restraints, Wandering

INTRODUCTION

Nurses caring for people with dementia frequently address safety issues, including falls and unsafe wandering. Safety concerns are usually heightened when people with dementia are in unfamiliar environments and when they have medical problems. Although physical restraints have been used in the past, healthcare professionals now recognize that restraints are rarely an appropriate intervention for ensuring safety. Nurses need to address safety issues as an important aspect of care for people with dementia.

In this chapter, you will learn:

1. How to assess fall risks in people with dementia
2. Interventions for preventing falls and fall-related injuries
3. How to avoid the use of restraints
4. How to address wandering

PREVENTING FALLS IN PEOPLE WITH DEMENTIA

People with dementia are at high risk for falls, and **half of the falls in people with dementia result in injury, including hip fractures**. Falls are usually attributed to a combination of risk conditions, which tend to be cumulative as dementia progresses. Nursing responsibilities include identifying and addressing conditions that increase the risk for falls or fall-related injuries. Interventions are implemented through the teamwork of many healthcare professionals, with nurses having lead roles.

Assessing Fall Risk

Institutional settings routinely incorporate evidence-based **fall-risk assessment tools** as an integral part of the nursing assessment and documentation, but these tools are not specifically for people with dementia. **Nurses need to add another layer to your fall-risk assessment** and identify any condition that poses a risk for falls in any individual patient. Box 14.1 lists conditions most often associated with increased risk for falls in people with moderate or advanced dementia.

BOX 14.1 CONDITIONS THAT INCREASE THE RISK FOR FALLS IN PEOPLE WITH MODERATE OR ADVANCED DEMENTIA

General Considerations
- New admission or transfer
- Fall(s) within past month
- Bladder and/or bowel incontinence
- Acute illness

Cognitive and Sensory Factors
- Depression
- Impaired judgment
- Lack of insight about limitations
- Communication impairments
- Visual or hearing impairment

Gait, Balance, and Mobility Factors
- Ambulatory but weak or debilitated
- Unable to use assistive devices properly
- Impaired balance or gait

Neuromotor Function
- Slow reflexes
- Neuromuscular rigidity

Behaviors
- Wandering
- Restless pacing
- Resistance to care
- Anxiety, agitation
- Sleep disturbances

Assess and document fall risks during the initial assessment and whenever the person's condition changes. This is especially important when caring for people whose mental status fluctuates, as is often the case with dementia and concomitant medical conditions.

Fast Facts

When caring for people with dementia, supplement standard assessment tools and document additional dementia-specific risks.

Addressing Fall Risks

Although it may be routine to fill out a fall-risk checklist in a patient's chart, the difficult—but essential—nursing responsibility is to address all the conditions that are amenable to interventions. Table 14.1 describes potentially reversible risk conditions and associated nursing actions to address them. Be proactive when caring for people who are cognitively compromised. For example, it may be appropriate to request a bedside sitter or companion caregivers, as they are becoming more widely available in hospital settings.

Fast Facts

Nurses have many opportunities to address conditions that are identified in fall-risk assessment tools.

◐ Clinical Snapshot

Mr. W is admitted with a primary diagnosis of aspiration pneumonia and secondary diagnoses of Parkinson's disease and advanced dementia. He usually walks with a walker and one assistant, but he has fallen several times during the past 6 months. He is very confused and frequently attempts to get out of bed. Family members tell you they can take turns staying at his bedside during the day, but they are unable to do so at night. You ask for orders for physical therapy and a request for a bedside companion to fill the hours when he will be unattended.

Table 14.1

Nursing Actions to Address Fall Risks

Risk Condition	Nursing Actions
Poor balance, impaired mobility, bed rest, muscular weakness	Assist as necessary to maintain the maximum level of safe mobility. Request physical therapy for evaluation and treatment. Provide range of motion exercise daily or as appropriate. Teach family and care partners about assisting with exercise and safe mobility. *For people being discharged to community settings:* Consider referral for physical therapy follow-up through home care agency for homebound people and in outpatient setting for people who are not homebound.
Adverse medication effects	Request pharmacy consult to review and advise about medications.
Unable to request help or use call system	Assign room near nursing station. Anticipate needs frequently, especially for toileting. Make sure all of the staff know that the person is unable to ask for help. Observe for nonverbal indicators of need and offer help. Arrange for bedside companion to observe, assist, and call for help. Use monitoring devices, such as pressure-activated pads with sound signals, and make sure that all the staff are aware of the need to respond quickly to alerting devices.
Lack of sturdy nonslip footwear	Make sure the person uses nonskid foot protectors or appropriate shoes or slippers during transfers and ambulation.
Unsafe bedside environment	Assess bedside environment for items that contribute to falls (including walkers, wheelchairs, and medical equipment) and move any items that pose risks for falls or injury.

(continued)

Table 14.1

Nursing Actions to Address Fall Risks (*continued*)

Risk Condition	Nursing Actions
Inadequate physical activity	Discharge instructions: Teach about importance of engaging in safe and enjoyable physical activities (e.g., mall walking, video or television programs, and games). Discharge instructions: Encourage participation in group activities for exercise (e.g., dancing, tai chi, walking clubs, Wii bowling, and other video-based programs).
Reduced vision	Make sure eyeglasses are clean and available and provide reminders or assistance if needed.
Unsafe home environment	Teach about a safe home environment: uncluttered, good lighting, no throw rugs, and no cords or other objects associated with tripping. Teach about bathroom safety equipment: grab bars, elevated toilet seat, and tub seat or shower chair. Consider referral for home evaluation by physical and occupational therapists as part of the discharge plan for patients returning home or to community settings.

Preventing Fall-Related Injuries

In addition to taking action to prevent falls, nurses are responsible for implementing interventions to reduce fractures and other injuries when falls do occur. For example, nurses can address **osteoporosis** (i.e., diminished bone density)—which occurs to some degree in all men and women by age 75 and increases the risk of fractures—through interventions such as:

- Finding out if the person has had screening tests such as bone mineral density to evaluate for osteoporosis
- Encouraging discussion with the primary care provider about medications for osteoporosis if the person has a history of fractures
- Teaching about the importance of weight-bearing exercise for 30 minutes daily

■ Teaching about adequate amounts of calcium (1,200–1,500 mg/day) and vitamin D (800–1,000 IU/day) in food or supplements

Another focus of nursing interventions is **addressing environmental conditions** that can cause cuts, bruises, bleeding, and other fall-related injuries. Examples of these interventions are:

■ Keeping the bed in the lowest position possible
■ Removing objects and furniture that can cause harm
■ Keeping the environment uncluttered and safe
■ Providing good lighting

Fast Facts

Incorporate information about health-promotion interventions for osteoporosis for prevention of fractures.

Clinical Snapshot

Mrs. O is 81 years old and is in the emergency room for evaluation of injuries sustained when she tripped at home. X-rays indicate she has no fractures, but she has a history of a fractured wrist 5 years ago. You encourage her to ask her doctor about osteoporosis and you teach her about a safe home environment.

PHYSICAL RESTRAINTS

The Centers for Medicare and Medicaid define a physical restraint as any **manual method, physical or mechanical device, or equipment that limits a person's movement of the body, head, or extremities freely**. Examples include hand mitts; elbow splints; full side rails; chairs with tabletops; and waist, vest, wrist, or leg restraints. Despite the common perception that physical restraints protect from falls, little evidence supports their effectiveness and more evidence shows their detrimental effects. Poor outcomes associated with physical restraints in people with dementia include:

■ Exacerbation of confusion
■ Increased agitation and anxiety
■ Increased risk of fall-related injury
■ Negative emotional responses, including fear, anger, resistance, and humiliation

- Physical deconditioning
- Decline in functioning
- Bruises, skin tears, pressure ulcers
- Urinary incontinence
- Constipation and fecal impaction
- Musculoskeletal injury (strains, contractures, limited range of motion)
- Strangulation or asphyxiation

Avoiding Restraints

Evidence-based information about the adverse effects of physical restraints and a focus on person-centered care for people with dementia have led to the development of "restraint-free" care in institutional settings. Interventions for avoiding restraints include all those discussed for fall prevention (Table 14.1) and interventions to address dementia-associated behaviors, as discussed in Chapter 11, Dementia-Associated Behaviors. Interventions related to invasive treatment devices include:

- Using the least invasive method to deliver care
- Repeatedly communicating about the purpose of the treatment in terms that the person can understand
- Protecting and camouflaging the device with clothing, protective sleeve, or temporary air splint
- Soliciting assistance from family, care partners, and activities staff to provide diversionary activities
- Discontinuing invasive treatments as soon as possible

Fast Facts

Physical restraints are not effective for reducing falls and are associated with many adverse effects, including increased risk for fall-related injuries.

WANDERING AND PACING

One of the major reasons for consideration of restraints is that people with dementia often exhibit wandering (i.e., frequent or excessive walking without an apparent destination) or pacing. Even though these behaviors may appear to be purposeless, people with dementia may be looking for ways to meet their physical or emotional needs.

Wandering and pacing also may be indicators of motor restlessness associated with adverse medication effects or medical conditions. Any of the following conditions can trigger wandering and pacing in a person with dementia:

- Physical discomfort (pain, hunger, thirst, or too hot or too cold)
- Physical need (finding a toilet)
- Need to change position (attempt at comfort or pain relief)
- Restlessness as adverse effect of medications (*akathisia*—severe motor restlessness due to antipsychotics or antidepressants—may look like persistent anxiety or aggressiveness)
- Stimulating effect of some drugs (caffeine, antidepressants)
- Anticholinergics can cause general feelings of restlessness
- Drugs may cause increased urge to urinate or defecate and may cause pacing
- Bowel or bladder disorders (urinary tract infections [UTI], constipation) may lead to pacing
- Medical conditions that can cause pacing and restlessness: depression, neuropathies, skin disorders, thyroid disease
- Dementia itself, depending on area of brain
- Overstimulation or understimulation (boredom)
- Believing they are elsewhere and need to do something (go to work, pick children up from school)
- Lack of exercise, need for physical activity
- Delayed reaction to overstimulation from the evening or day before

Addressing Wandering and Pacing

Address conditions that trigger wandering and pacing by applying the interventions discussed in Chapter 11, Dementia-Associated Behaviors, for dementia-associated behaviors. Additional interventions, specific to addressing wandering and pacing in hospital settings, include:

- Making referrals for physical therapy for interventions to support safe walking
- Providing appropriate supervision (e.g., placing them in a room that allows for maximum observation, frequent checking, and requesting assistance of companions or specialized staff)
- Using movement-detection devices to alert staff (e.g., pressure pads with audible signal)
- Reducing environmental triggers (avoiding rooms near high levels of activity, keeping the person's street clothing and shoes out of sight)

- Providing orientation cues and frequent reminders (e.g., "You'll be staying in the hospital until you are better")
- Distracting the person's attention

Fast Facts

Nurses need to identify conditions and needs that trigger wandering and pacing and recognize that the behaviors are an attempt to meet a physical or emotional need.

RESOURCES

Alzheimer's Association

https://www.alz.org

- Reports and recommendations on falls, wandering, and physical restraints

American Geriatrics Society, Clinical Practice Guideline on Prevention of Falls in Older Persons

https://www.americangeriatrics.org

Hartford Institute for Geriatric Nursing

https://www.consultgerirn.org

- Fall Risk Assessment, *Try This*, Issue 5, and video illustrating application of assessment tool
- Avoiding Restraints in Older Adults with Dementia, *Try This*, Issue D1, article and video
- Wandering in Hospitalized Older Adults, *Try This*, Issue D6, article and video
- Evidence-based guidelines on use of physical restraints with elderly patients
- Nursing standards of practice protocol: Fall prevention

15

Nursing Assessment and Management of Pain in People With Dementia

INTRODUCTION

Pain management is one of the most important aspects of nursing care for people with dementia because, compared with people who have no cognitive impairment, people with dementia have higher rates of pain and are less likely to have it treated adequately. Nurses are the healthcare professionals who are best able to assess and manage pain to improve comfort, functioning, and quality of life for people with dementia. This chapter provides an overview of nursing responsibilities associated with the unique aspects of pain in people with dementia.

In this chapter, you will learn:

1. Unique manifestations of pain in people with dementia
2. Nursing assessment of pain in people with dementia
3. Pharmacological management
4. Nonpharmacological interventions
5. Cultural considerations related to pain

UNIQUE MANIFESTATIONS OF PAIN IN PEOPLE WITH DEMENTIA

Dementia does not alter the physiological processes involved with the transmission of pain; however, it can affect the person's perception and expression of pain, particularly during moderate and later stages. For example, **people with dementia who have limited verbal communication are likely to manifest their pain behaviorally through aggression or agitation** (Nowak, Neumann-Podezaska, Tobis, & Wieczorowska-Tobis, 2019). Consequently, pain is often unrecognized, untreated, or inappropriately treated with psychotropics rather than analgesics. Pain assessment in people with dementia is further complicated when there is a combination of acute and chronic conditions, as is often the case. Thus, pain assessment and management are ongoing and dynamic processes requiring nursing leadership and input from all care providers, with the recognition that expressions of pain may change frequently during the course of dementia.

People with mild or moderate dementia may be able to accurately report pain if nurses elicit information through techniques such as the following:

- Offer examples of words that communicate pain and discomfort: hurting, sore, achy, tender, and ouch.
- Ask "Are you hurting or uncomfortable in any way?"
- If you suspect that an area is painful or uncomfortable, point or use gentle touch, and ask "How does your _____ [knee, head, stomach] feel now?"
- When people with dementia report pain or discomfort in a specific area, ask them to point to the area to verify the location (e.g., they may say their head hurts, but point to their shoulder when asked to verify).

In addition, nurses can obtain information from the person's family and care partners. Ask if there are particular words or behaviors the person typically uses to communicate about pain or discomfort.

As the ability to self-report about experiences of pain diminishes during the course of dementia, **nurses and care partners must increasingly rely on observations and other sources of information to assess pain**. Review the patient's chart for information about chronic or recurring conditions that may cause pain, such as arthritis, fibromyalgia, back pain, postherpetic neuralgia, and diabetic neuropathies. Observe for indicators of pain or discomfort such as the examples listed in Table 15.1. A recent review of studies found strong evidence for restlessness (agitation), rubbing, guarding, rigidity, and physical aggression as reliable indicators of pain in cognitively impaired people (Strand et al., 2019).

Table 15.1

Indicator	Examples
Behaviors	Agitation, irritability, increased confusion, change in mental status
Overall movements	Restlessness, shifting positions, repetitive hand movements, rubbing or massaging affected area
Movement of extremities	Guarding, diminished weight-bearing ability, limited range of motion
Physical changes	Redness, swelling, elevated temperature
Response during activities or treatments	Resistance, protective actions, tightening, combativeness
Recent falls or other injuries	Bruises, burns, wounds, skin tears
Activities of daily living	Poor appetite, increased dependency, changes in functioning
Psychosocial function	Mood swings, withdrawal from usual social activities, agitation, changes in relationships

In the words of a nursing assistant:

> It is hard to explain how you can read that there is pain in her face, but the fact that she was rubbing and she didn't look as happy as usual . . . we got the doctor to see her and she has bad knees and I try to say they be swollen, so she on regular pain pills now. (Watson, 2019, p. 553)

Fast Facts

People with dementia do communicate about pain, but they may do so nonverbally, indirectly, verbally but imprecisely, or behaviorally.

NURSING ASSESSMENT OF PAIN IN PEOPLE WITH DEMENTIA

Pain, considered the "fourth vital sign," is usually assessed according to universally recognized scales, such as "on a scale of 1 to 10, with 10 being the most severe level." During early stages, people with dementia usually maintain some ability to self-report and respond to a simple verbal scale such as those commonly in use. However, **as their communication abilities become more impaired, they are less able to self-report and care providers need to use assessment tools based on observation.** The Pain Assessment Checklist for Seniors with Limited Ability to Communicate–II (PACSLAC–II) is an easy-to-use and evidence-based tool for clinical settings that identifies and assesses pain in people with dementia (see Exhibit 15.1; Hadjistavropoulos et al., 2018). The Resources section at the end of this chapter lists websites for information about this and other tools that document assessment observations.

Exhibit 15.1

The Pain Assessment Checklist for Seniors With Limited Ability to Communicate–II (PACSLAC–II)

Date of Assessment: _____ Time: _____	Check if present
Facial Expressions	
1. Grimacing	
2. Tighter face	
3. Pain expression	
4. Increased eye movement	
5. Wincing	
6. Opening mouth	
7. Creasing forehead	
8. Lowered eyebrows or frowning	
9. Raised cheeks, narrowing of the eyes or squinting	
10. Wrinkled nose and raised upper lip	
11. Eyes closing	
Verbalizations and Vocalizations	
12. Crying	
13. A specific sound for pain (e.g., "ow," "ouch")	
14. Moaning and groaning	
15. Grunting	
16. Gasping or breathing loudly	
Body Movements	
17. Flinching or pulling away	
18. Thrashing	
19. Refusing to move	
20. Moving slow	
21. Guarding sore area	

22. Rubbing or holding sore area	
23. Limping	
24. Clenched fist	
25. Going into foetal position	
26. Stiff or rigid	
27. Shaking or trembling	
Changes in Interpersonal Interactions	
28. Not wanting to be touched	
29. Not allowing people near	
Changes in Activity Patterns or Routines	
30. Decreased activity	
Mental Status Changes	
31. Are there mental status changes that are due to pain and are not explained by another condition (e.g., delirium due to medication, etc.)?	
TOTAL SCORE (Add up checkmarks)	

Source: Reproduced with permission from Thomas Hadjistavropoulos, PhD, RD Psych, ABPP. Retrieved from *http://www.geriatricpain.org/*. (The PACSLAC–II may not be reproduced without permission. For permission to reproduce the PACSLAC–II contact the worldwide copyright holders thomas.hadjistavropoulos@uregina.ca).

Fast Facts

When assessing pain in people who cannot reliably self-report, nurses use assessment observations as detailed in Table 15.1 and Exhibit 15.1.

🌀 Clinical Snapshot

Mrs. G is admitted to the hospital for heart failure and has additional diagnoses of dementia and osteoarthritis. Nurses document that she does not respond accurately when asked to rate her pain on a scale of 1 to 10. Using the PACSLAC–II, they document the following indicators of pain when they assist her with transferring to the bedside commode: grimacing, overall muscle tightening, and not wanting to be touched. When Mrs. G.'s daughter visits, they find out that Mrs. G. had been taking over-the-counter analgesics for her osteoarthritis, but she was not receiving these in the hospital.

PHARMACOLOGICAL MANAGEMENT OF PAIN

Implementing effective treatments for pain and its underlying causes is a multidisciplinary process involving teamwork with nurses, physicians, pharmacists, and all care providers. Pain management involves pharmacological and nonpharmacological interventions and ongoing assessment of both the effectiveness and adverse effects of these interventions. In addition, when caring for people with dementia, it is important to recognize that **expressions of pain or discomfort may be due to physical needs** related to hunger, thirst, need for assistance with toileting, or environmental conditions (e.g., noisy, overstimulating, hot or cold temperatures). Ultimately, identify and address basic physical and emotional needs as much as possible.

Dementia experts emphasize that **unrecognized and untreated pain is a common cause of challenging behaviors**. In many situations, the connection between pain and behavior is not obvious. For example, when the person with dementia and limited verbal abilities experiences persistent or intermittent pain from chronic conditions, apply all the assessment guidelines discussed in this chapter and determine whether chronic pain is potentially a cause of challenging behaviors or whether it affects functioning or quality of life for the person with dementia. If there is reason to suspect the person is experiencing pain or discomfort from a chronic condition, a trial of analgesic medications may be warranted following the guidelines in Exhibit 15.2.

Exhibit 15.2

Guidelines for Pharmacological Management of Persistent Pain in Older Adults With Dementia

General Guidelines

- Analgesics should be initiated at low doses and titrated upward for optimum pain relief and minimal adverse effects.
- Initial and ongoing evaluation of therapeutic and adverse effects is essential.
- Regular, rather than as needed, doses are preferable for people who are cognitively impaired and cannot request medications appropriately.

- Medications should be provided around the clock for people with continuous pain.
- Pharmacologic interventions should be combined with nonpharmacologic approaches to enhance effectiveness.
  - Nonpharmacological interventions for persistent pain include heat, exercise, physical therapy, acupuncture, and massage
  - Psychosocial interventions for persistent pain include music, guided imagery, cognitive-behavioral therapy, mindfulness-based meditation

Guidelines related to specific medication types

- Acetaminophen (Tylenol) for musculoskeletal conditions (e.g., osteoarthritis and lower back pain); 650–1,000 mg every 6–8 hours with lower doses or precautions as appropriate (e.g., hepatic insufficiency, when combined with opioids)
- Nonsteroidal anti-inflammatory drugs (NSAIDs) for chronic inflammatory conditions (e.g., rheumatoid arthritis) or short-term relief of musculoskeletal conditions; caution or contraindicated with renal insufficiency, gastropathy, hypertension, cardiovascular disease; contraindicated with anticoagulants or low-dose aspirin.
- For localized pain, use topical analgesics (e.g., capsaicin, lidocaine, camphor-menthol combinations, NSAIDs).
- Begin trial with opioid analgesics with caution if other interventions are ineffective or if significant risk of serious adverse effects from NSAIDs or acetaminophen. Establish clearly defined goals and discontinue if goals are not achieved; assess, prevent, and treat constipation and other adverse effects.
- Use adjuvant drugs such as antidepressants, anticonvulsants (e.g., gabapentin [Neurontin], pregabalin [Lyrica]) alone or in combination with analgesics for certain conditions (e.g., fibromyalgia, neuropathic pain); evaluate anticholinergic or sedating adverse effects.
- Use corticosteroids for rheumatic and autoimmune conditions (rheumatoid arthritis, giant cell arteritis).

Fast Facts

Agitation in people with moderate or advanced dementia may be caused by persistent pain.

Clinical Snapshot

Mr. P has advanced dementia and has a history of arthritis in both knees and hips. He rarely gets out of the chair, even though he has good mobility and balance. When nursing assistants encourage him to walk to the dining room, he becomes combative and yells, "No, no!" After he begins taking acetaminophen 750 mg every 6 hours, he is less agitated and willing to walk several times a day.

NONPHARMACOLOGICAL INTERVENTIONS

Many nonpharmacological interventions are effective for persistent pain and these may be particularly helpful for people with mild or moderate dementia. Nurses can suggest the following interventions that can enhance pain management:

- Yoga
- Reiki
- Aquatherapy
- Massage
- Therapeutic touch
- Acupuncture
- Meditation
- Visual or auditory distraction (calming music, scenes of nature)

Suggest a referral for physical therapy for pain-management interventions that might be covered by health insurance. Community centers and health centers may also offer resources for many of these interventions; sometimes they are covered by insurance or provided at a discounted rate.

Fast Facts

Nurses have many opportunities to suggest nonpharmacological interventions for persistent pain in people with dementia, such as

(continued)

(continued)

physical therapy for musculoskeletal conditions. People with mild dementia are capable of engaging in self-care activities such as yoga or meditation.

🄲 Clinical Snapshot

Mr. R, who has mild dementia, is being discharged from rehabilitation following recovery from total hip replacement surgery. His wife asks if there are other things he can do to address his discomfort and maintain his walking and balance. You suggest they both consider joining the weekly tai chi classes that are held at the senior center where they have gone for meals.

CULTURAL CONSIDERATIONS RELATED TO PAIN

Cultural factors can significantly influence the way people experience, express, and manage their pain. Examples of cultural variations are as following:

- Some cultural groups are traditionally very stoic whereas others may be very outspoken
- Some describe pain in terms of diverse body symptoms
- Some consider that bearing pain is a virtue or sign of strength
- Some believe that pain and suffering can be relieved by prayer and the laying on of hands

Nursing assessment of pain includes consideration of cultural variations while also avoiding stereotypes.

References

Hadjistavropoulos, T., Browne, M. E., Prkachin, K. M., Taati, B., Ashraf, A., & Mihailidis, A. (2018). Pain in severe dementia: A comparison of a fine-grained assessment approach to an observational checklist designed for clinical settings. *European Journal of Pain, 22*(5), 915–925. doi:10.1002/ejp.1177

Nowak, T., Neumann-Podezaska, A., Tobis, S., & Wieczorowska-Tobis, K. (2019). Characteristics of pharmacological pain treatment in older nursing home residents. *Journal of Pain Research, 25*(12), 1083–1089. doi:10.2147/JPR.S192587

Strand, L, Gendrosen, K. F., Lein, R. K., Laekeman, M., Lobbezoo, F., Defrin, R., & Husebo, B. S. (2019). Body movements as pain indicators in older people with cognitive impairment: A systematic review. *European Journal of Pain, 23*(4), 669–684. doi:10.1002/ejp.1344

Watson, J. (2019). Developing the Senses Framework to support relationship-centered care for people with advanced dementia until the end of life in care homes. *Dementia, 18*(2), 545–566. doi:10.1177/1471301216682880

RESOURCES

American Geriatrics Society, Foundation for Health in Aging

https://www.healthinaging.org

- Pain in Dementia: Family and Caregivers Guide to Assessment and Treatment

Geriatric Pain

https://www.geriatricpain.org

https://www.seepainmoreclearly.org/resources

Hartford Institute for Geriatric Nursing
www.consultgerirn.org

- Assessing Pain in Persons With Dementia, *Try This*, Issue D2, and video illustrating application of assessment tool
- Using Pain-Rating Scales in Older Adults, *Try This*, Issue 7, and video illustrating application of assessment tools
- Assessment of Nociceptive Versus Neuropathic Pain in Older Adults, *Try This*, Issue SP1

VI

Broader Aspects of Care for People With Dementia

16

Self-Neglect and Elder Abuse of People With Dementia

INTRODUCTION

Dementia increases the risk for elder abuse, defined as an act or lack of appropriate action that (a) occurs within any relationship in which there is an expectation of trust or dependence and (b) causes harm or distress to an older person. Self-neglect is a type of elder abuse that does not involve a relationship with another person and is defined as behavior of an elderly person that threatens his or her own health or safety.

In this chapter, you will learn:

1. An overview of elder abuse and people with dementia
2. Nursing assessment for elder abuse in the person with dementia
3. Cultural considerations
4. Nursing assessment of caregivers
5. Roles of nurses in elder abuse situations
6. Adult protective service laws

OVERVIEW: ELDER ABUSE AND PEOPLE WITH DEMENTIA

Dementia increases the risk for self-neglect and elder abuse and neglect. Be alert to this possibility and take appropriate actions. Elder abuse occurs under any of the following circumstances:

- Physical abuse, sexual abuse, emotional or psychological abuse, and financial or material exploitation: A caregiver or other responsible person performs acts that cause or create a serious risk of harm to a vulnerable older adult.
- Neglect or abandonment: Caregiver or another responsible person fails to satisfy the elder's basic needs or to protect the elder from harm.
- Self-neglect: The behaviors of older adults threaten their health or safety.

Dementia characteristics associated with increased risk for elder abuse are summarized in Table 16.1.

Table 16.1

Dementia Characteristics Associated With Increased Risk for Elder Abuse	
Dementia Characteristic	**Associated Increased Risk**
Difficulty managing financial affairs	Financial exploitation
Limited insight and awareness	Decreased ability to self-report
Impaired short-term memory	Decreased ability to relate details
Cognitive impairment	Questionable credibility of information
Social isolation	Increased risk for self-neglect
Dementia-related difficult behaviors	Increased risk for abuse or neglect by caregiver
Functional dependency	Increased risk for self-neglect or neglect by caregiver
Long-term and progressive course	Increased risk for abusive behaviors by caregivers

In the words of a family member concerned about self-neglect:

> The house started to decline. He did not clean. It smelled horrible inside the house. He did not turn the stove on, it was freezing cold, and he had no lights on. . . . I was worried sick; it was exhausting. (Rasmussen, Hellzen, Stordal, & Enmarker, 2019)

NURSING ASSESSMENT OF THE PERSON WITH DEMENTIA

Be on the alert for indicators of abuse and neglect when caring for people with dementia. Recognize that elder abuse is usually well hidden, sometimes for a long time, and information may be purposefully withheld. Clues to elder abuse might first be noted when a vulnerable older person is seen in an ED or admitted to a hospital. Nurses may identify the indicators of elder abuse listed in Table 16.2 during a usual patient assessment, but when these conditions are identified, the pieces of the puzzle need to be put together to detect elder abuse or neglect.

Fast Facts

It is imperative to be alert for indicators of elder abuse or neglect when assessing people who have dementia.

Clinical Snapshot

When Mrs. P was admitted for a hip fracture, the nursing assessment noted that she had very poor hygiene, matted and oily hair, multiple bruises on her trunk and upper arms, and long toenails that curled under her toes. The nurse discussed this with Mrs. P's doctor and asked for further assessment of nutritional status and a referral for social services.

Table 16.2

Nursing Assessment for Indicators of Elder Abuse or Neglect

Assessment Parameter	What to Look for
Hydration	Dry mucous membranes, dry mouth, poor skin turgor over sternum and abdomen, concentrated urine
Nutrition	Dry, fissured, cracked lips; tongue and mucous membranes inflamed, ulcerated, or with white patches
Laboratory indicators for nutritional deficiency	Anemia; low serum glucose, sodium, potassium, ferritin, folate, or vitamin B_{12}; serum albumin level less than 5.5 g/dL; cholesterol levels less than 160 mg/dL; total iron-binding capacity less than 250 mcg/dL
Skin	Leg or pressure ulcers, poor wound healing
Injuries from falls, accidents, or abuse	Swelling; limited range of motion; evidence of burns from stoves, cigarettes, or hot water; marks from cuts, bites, or punctures

(continued)

Table 16.3

Nursing Assessment for Indicators of Elder Abuse or Neglect (*continued*)

Assessment Parameter	What to Look for
Bruise patterns characteristic of abuse	Bruises that reflect the shape of objects; bruises on the trunk, face, head, or both upper arms; bruises at various stages of healing (e.g., yellow, blue, red, purple)
Overall appearance	Weight loss, poor muscle tone, decreased strength, frailty, poor hygiene, edema, extremely long nails (including long toenails that interfere with mobility)
Indicators of excessive amounts of drugs or alcohol	Excessive somnolence, clouded mentation, slurred speech, staggering gait, difficulty walking, poor balance
Mood	Depressed, listless, apathetic, agitated

CULTURAL CONSIDERATIONS

Cultural influences can affect all the following aspects of elder abuse in people with dementia:

- Perception that people with dementia do not feel the effects of elder abuse
- Perception that people with dementia-related behaviors may "deserve" behaviors that otherwise would be viewed as abusive
- Perception that actions of family caregivers who are stressed and well-intentioned are not abusive

While it is important to consider cultural variations that influence perceptions of elder abuse in people with dementia, nurses have legal and ethical obligations to identify indicators of elder abuse and initiate appropriate interventions.

NURSING ASSESSMENT OF CAREGIVERS

In addition to assessing the person with dementia for the indicators listed in Table 16.2, **look for clues in the broader caregiver situation**. Nurses have many opportunities to identify indicators of abuse or neglect in statements and actions of caregivers when they are visiting the person with dementia. Caregiving itself does not cause elder abuse; however, it can lead to abuse when those assuming the caregiving role are incapable of doing so due to life stresses, pathologic characteristics, personality characteristics, insufficient resources, or lack of understanding of the older adult's condition. Caregivers who perpetrate abuse often exhibit some of the same risk factors associated with abused elders, particularly if the caregivers themselves are older adults.

Caregiver factors associated with elder abuse:

- Poor health
- Cognitive impairment
- Social isolation
- Dependency
- Coresidence
- Poor interpersonal relations with the dependent elder

It is not unusual to have a mutually neglectful or abusive situation when an older married couple have several of the psychosocial risk factors just identified and are, in addition, socially isolated.

Fast Facts

A key indicator of elder abuse or neglect can be obtained through observation and documentation of caregivers.

◌ Clinical Snapshot

Mrs. E is in the cardiac intensive care unit with a diagnosis of myocardial infarction and she has a concomitant diagnosis of dementia. Upon admission, her personal appearance was unkempt and her blood tests indicate that she is malnourished. When her husband comes to visit, you note that his appearance is unkempt, his clothes are baggy, and he has trouble remembering and processing information. You request social service involvement for further assessment.

ROLES OF NURSES IN ELDER ABUSE SITUATIONS

A primary role for nurses is to assess for indicators of abuse and follow institutional policy for reporting suspected abuse to the public agency responsible for implementing adult protective service laws. Adult protective service laws do not require reporters to *know* whether abuse or neglect has occurred, but merely to report it if they *suspect* its occurrence. The responsibility for problem verification rests with the public agency charged with implementing the law, not with the reporter or referral source. Protocols and screening tools for elder mistreatment and abuse are available through the websites listed in the Resources section at the end of this chapter.

When elder abuse or neglect is caused by caregiver stress, initiate a referral for social services. Nurses also can incorporate the following interventions when they talk with care partners:

- Encourage families to reevaluate the demands of the situation and consider resources for support and assistance.
- Emphasize that care partners need to take care of themselves.
- Encourage care partners to find resources for delegating some of their responsibilities.
- Facilitate communication among all the decision makers, including the primary care provider, the older adult (if appropriate), and family members who are responsible for care.
- Suggest participation in educational or support groups.
- Identify patient's needs for skilled care and initiate referrals as appropriate (e.g., a recent fall may qualify the person for physical therapy or a change in medication may qualify the person for skilled nursing at home).
- Suggest types of medical equipment, disposable supplies, and assistive devices to improve function and safety for the elder and ease caregiver burden (e.g., caregivers may respond positively to suggestions about using grab bars for preventing falls in the bathroom).

ADULT PROTECTIVE SERVICE LAWS

All states have adult protective services laws that address elder abuse and neglect. Although these laws differ, some common elements are pertinent to nurses:

- Reporting suspected abuse is mandatory in most states, and nurses are the healthcare workers most commonly identified as mandatory reporters.
- Most state laws protect the confidentiality of reports and the identity of all people involved in making them.
- Most reporting laws provide immunity for mandatory reporters, so nurses who act in good faith can report suspected cases without fear of liability.

- Penalties for failure to report include a charge of a misdemeanor, financial penalty, civil liability, or notification of the state licensing board.

Fast Facts

Become familiar with adult protective service laws that apply to a clinical practice setting and follow protocols for reporting elder abuse and neglect.

Reference

Rasmussen, H., Hellzen, O., Stordal, E., & Enmarker, I. (2019). Family caregivers experiences of the pre-diagnostic stage in frontotemporal dementia. *Geriatric Nursing, 40*, 246–251. doi:10.1016/j.gerinurse.2018.10.006

RESOURCES

Hartford Institute for Geriatric Nursing

https://consultgeri.org

- Elder Mistreatment and Abuse protocol
- Elder Mistreatment Assessment, *Try This*, Issue 15 and video illustrating application of the assessment tool

National Center on Elder Abuse

https://ncea.acl.gov

17

Ethical and Legal Issues

INTRODUCTION

Supporting the rights of the person with dementia is one of the greatest challenges—and a core aspect—of person-centered care. During the course of dementia, many questions arise about the person's rights to carry out activities that become risky or unsafe because of cognitive impairments. These issues typically arise during mild and moderate dementia and continue until people with dementia are no longer able to participate in decisions about their care. During advanced dementia, additional issues arise related to decisions about medical interventions and goals of care, as discussed in Chapter 9, Caring for the Person With Advanced Dementia. Nurses can address these issues by considering ethical and legal guidelines as discussed in this chapter.

In this chapter, you will learn:

1. Ethical issues related to the rights of people with dementia
2. Nursing considerations related to decisional capacity in people with dementia
3. Legal documents that protect the rights of people with dementia
4. Nursing responsibilities related to advance directives

ETHICAL ISSUES RELATED TO THE RIGHTS OF PEOPLE WITH DEMENTIA

A common misperception is that someone with a diagnosis of dementia does not have the ability to make decisions. This misperception is reinforced by ageist perceptions of older adults as incompetent. In reality, the **decision-making abilities of people with dementia change gradually and usually are well maintained until later stages**. Even during the moderate stage, people with dementia typically maintain the ability to be involved with decision-making. When their decision-making abilities are significantly impaired, they increasingly rely on others to protect them from harm and advocate for their wishes.

All competent adults have the right to direct their own lives as long as their actions do not infringe on the rights of others, but they can lose this right if they do not have **decisional capacity.** People who have decisional capacity must be able to do all the following:

- Understand relevant information.
- Demonstrate comprehension of the information.
- Apply the information to one's own situation.
- Consider alternatives and the associated consequences.
- Communicate the decision to others.
- Take appropriate actions to implement the decision.

In the ideal situation, **the person has all legal documents in order and has supportive family and care partners who make decisions consistent with the wishes of the person with dementia.** In reality, however, ethical issues often arise because of a lack of appropriate legal documents, disagreements among surrogate decision makers, or resistance on the part of the person with dementia. In these situations, nurses and other healthcare providers are likely to be involved with decisions involving freedom versus safety for the person with dementia. Sometimes, the decisions relate to a **situation that is not harmful but poses a risk for harm**. These situations involve weighing the person's freedom and safety against probable or possible harm. Many of these issues are associated with daily activities and there is loss of roles and responsibilities that the person carried out independently for many years, as illustrated by the following examples:

- Driving a vehicle
- Living alone
- Refusing or resisting assistance with activities of daily living
- Cooking independently, even when the person frequently burns food
- Managing medications independently, even when it is not done reliably

- Refusing or resisting a move to a safer environment
- Refusing or resisting medical care
- Managing finances independently
- Walking independently, even with unsafe mobility
- Going outside one's home, even when the person is likely to get lost
- Smoking independently, even with the risk of fires

Fast Facts

Address decisions about issues related to daily activities by suggesting referrals for appropriate healthcare professionals and facilitating communication among all team members.

In the words of a family caregiver:

> She was able to go places that she was familiar with . . . and then she did it alone until one day, the police came when they found her wandering. How much do you allow them to do because on the one hand, you do not want them to be shut in beyond what is necessary but you do not want to risk it? (Truglio-Lonmdrigan & Slyer, 2019, p. 261)

ASSESSING DECISIONAL CAPACITY

These issues are addressed, in part, by **assessing the decisional capacity of the person with dementia, which is usually done by several healthcare professionals**, including nurses. In addition, nurses can facilitate referrals for the following healthcare professionals in Table 17.1.

Table 17.1

Reasons for Referrals	
Healthcare Professional	**Reason for Referral**
Occupational therapist	Assessment and rehabilitation services related to driving and other activities that may be risky
Physical therapist	Assessment and therapy for balance and mobility
Speech therapist	Assessment and interventions related to memory, cognition, and communication
Psychologist or social worker	Assessment and interventions to address resistance, conflicts, and coping
Social worker or geriatric care manager	Referrals for legal and financial professionals who specialize in eldercare issues

Decisional capacity is usually determined in relation to a particular situation, and it differs from **competency**, which is a legal term for the ability to fulfill one's roles and handle one's affairs in a responsible manner.

Nurses are involved with the assessment of decisional capacity when signatures are required for procedures and at many other times when they care for people with dementia. Consider the following when discussing decisions about care:

- People with mild and moderate dementia usually retain some decision-making capacity.
- Make arrangements if the person would like to involve other people in the discussion.
- Adapt your communication to the person's abilities; reinforce verbal with written information.
- Present the information in the most understandable terms.
- Allow time for the person to consider the information.
- Encourage the person to ask questions
- Obtain feedback to assess the person's understanding.
- Discuss the information ahead of time with trusted family members or surrogate decision makers and plan the best way to involve the person with dementia.
- Address conditions that can interfere with communication (e.g., ensuring that a hearing-impaired person uses his or her hearing aid).
- Plan discussions as much as possible when the person is rested, alert, and comfortable.
- When you have questions about the person's ability, ask another nurse to reassess at another time.
- If appropriate, involve other healthcare professionals.

One of the key roles of nurses in assessing decisional capacity is requesting evaluations from other healthcare professionals when the situation is unclear or when conflicts arise. This is especially important when major decisions are being made that affect the person's right to self-determination.

Fast Facts

Nurses have key roles in assessing decisional capacity and in facilitating referrals for other healthcare professionals (e.g., geriatricians, psychologists, psychiatrists, and social workers).

ESSENTIAL LEGAL DOCUMENTS

One of the most important aspects of caring for people with dementia is ensuring that legal documents are in place before issues arise about competency or decisional capacity. The Alzheimer's Association and dementia experts emphasize executing these legal documents as soon as the diagnosis has been made. Even when cognitive abilities are compromised, people with dementia may be capable of executing legal documents as long as they are able to understand the issues and communicate their intentions. Legal documents most pertinent to healthcare situations are the durable power of attorney for healthcare, living wills, and medical directives.

Durable Power of Attorney for Healthcare

A durable power of attorney for healthcare is **a legally binding document that takes effect whenever someone—for any reason—cannot provide informed consent for healthcare treatment decisions.** Because this document authorizes a surrogate decision maker (also called a healthcare proxy) to represent the person during any time of incapacity, it is often considered the most important legal document. A durable power of attorney for healthcare must be initiated when the person is competent, and it takes effect only when the person is incapacitated. Nurses are responsible for documenting information about the person's legally appointed surrogate decision makers and for including them in discussions and decisions about care.

The primary responsibility of the surrogate decision maker is to make and support decisions consistent with the wishes of the person with dementia. Ideally, these wishes have been documented in advance directives, and it is imperative that the healthcare proxy have a copy of all advance directives and periodically discuss the person's wishes. Even when the wishes are documented, these decisions are not always clear, and the surrogate decision maker may experience emotional turmoil about the decisions. Nurses often assume advisory roles in clarifying information and supporting the healthcare power of attorney when decisions are difficult.

If this legal document has not been executed, spouses, adult children, and other close relatives often assume decision-making responsibilities for the person with dementia. When conflicts arise among those who assume decision-making responsibilities and the person with dementia is not capable of making these decisions, more restrictive legal actions, such as guardianship, may be necessary. When nurses are aware of conflicts about decisions, they need to document this information and discuss this with other members of the healthcare team.

Fast Facts

Nurses provide information and support for surrogate decision makers.

⟳ Clinical Snapshot

Mrs. H's cardiologist has scheduled surgery for a pacemaker, and you are responsible for obtaining informed consent. Mrs. H has advanced dementia and her daughter, who is her surrogate decision maker, tells you she is not sure if her mother would want to have this done because she always said, "When it's my time, God will take me and I don't want any doctors or anyone else interfering with that plan." You give the daughter written information about the risks and benefits of the procedure, and you arrange for her to discuss this with the doctor.

Living Wills

Living wills are **advance directives allowing people to specify the type of medical treatment they would want or not want** if they become incapacitated as a result of terminal illness. These documents affirm the right of a person to refuse treatment, but they do not always specify the particular type of treatment that can be refused. They can document the person's preferences about pain management, organ donation, place of death, and specific treatments he or she would want to receive. Living wills apply only when the person is terminally ill, and this may be difficult to determine, particularly during advanced dementia (as discussed in Chapter 9, Caring for the Person With Advanced Dementia).

Medical Directives

A do-not-resuscitate (DNR) order is a very specific type of advance directive that compels healthcare providers to refrain from cardiopulmonary resuscitation if the person is no longer breathing and has no heartbeat. Some states allow variations of the DNR order, with the most common one being Comfort Care DNR (also called DNR-Comfort Care, CC/DNR, or Comfort Care Only DNR). These legal documents direct healthcare professionals to provide designated comfort care measures but not resuscitative therapies. In addition to addressing DNR interventions, medical directives can address specific interventions, such as antibiotics, food and nutrition, and admission to the hospital. These documents should be reviewed periodically, especially during advanced dementia.

RESPONSIBILITIES OF NURSES RELATED TO ADVANCE DIRECTIVES

Nurses have essential roles related to advance directives for people with dementia who have decisional capacity, including all the following:

- Being knowledgeable about pertinent state laws related to advance directives
- Teaching patients about advance directives
- Encouraging patients to execute such documents if they have not done so
- Encouraging patients to review and update their advance directives whenever their situation or that of their surrogate decision maker changes
- Assuring that advance directives are available in patient charts
- Communicating with other professionals about a patient's advance directives
- Documenting conversations about advance directives in patient charts

From an ethical perspective, advance directives provide a foundation for respecting the autonomy of the person with dementia when that person can no longer be actively engaged in decisions about his or her care.

Fast Facts

Nurses initiate discussions of advance directives when they care for people with dementia, document these discussions, and ensure that all pertinent documents are available for all healthcare professionals.

In the words of a person with dementia:

> I don't think anybody else should be involved in it except myself. I don't want any of my so-called family to be making decisions for me. (Xanthopoulou & McCabe, 2019, p. 7)

In the words of a family caregiver:

> What medical treatment do you continue? What about current medications for current conditions? Do you continue to do those? Is there a point where it does not make sense anymore? (Truglio-Londrigan & Slyer, 2019)

References

Truglio-Londrigan, M., & Slyer, J. (2019). Caregiver decisions along the Alzheimer's disease trajectory. *Geriatric Nursing, 40*, 257–263. doi:10.1016/j.gerinurse.2018.10.015

Xanthopoulou, P., & McCabe, R. (2019). Subjective experiences of cognitive decline and receiving a diagnosis of dementia: Qualitative interviews with people recently diagnosed in memory clinics in the UK. *BMJ Open, 9*(8), e026071. doi:10.1035/bmjopen-2018-026071

RESOURCES

Aging with Dignity

https://www.agingwithdignity.org

- Information about advance directives

Hartford Institute for Geriatric Nursing

https://consultgeri.org

- Decision Making and Dementia, *Try This,* Issue D9

18

Needs of Caregivers of People With Dementia

INTRODUCTION

As discussed throughout this book, nurses who care for people with dementia address many dementia-related issues during the course of usual care. In addition to addressing the many ways in which dementia influences the daily care of patients with dementia, nurses address the many ways in which this chronic condition affects the patients and their care partners over the long term. This may be especially evident when you develop a discharge plan and when family members and other care partners discuss their concerns with you. Although social workers are primarily responsible for addressing these needs, families of people with dementia often see nurses as a primary source of advice and guidance about dementia-related concerns. Thus, nurses are in key positions to teach about resources that address the needs of people with dementia and their care partners. This chapter provides an overview of the types of resources that you need to be aware of so you can holistically address the dementia-related needs of your patients and their care partners as an integral part of your care plan.

In this chapter, you will learn:

1. Resources for people with dementia and their caregivers' needs
2. Resources for assistance with care
3. Adult day centers
4. Residential care for people with dementia
5. Hospice and palliative care services

RESOURCES FOR PEOPLE WITH DEMENTIA AND THEIR CAREGIVERS

A relatively simple intervention is to teach about the Alzheimer's Association, which provides numerous resources that are available online and through local chapters everywhere in the United States. This resource can be "one-stop shopping" for information and referral through their helpline at 800-272-3900. If the person resists your suggestion because of the word "Alzheimer's," you can emphasize the association addresses needs of people with "related dementias" and "memory impairments" and is an excellent source of information for anyone dealing with similar issues. In addition, as part of the discharge plan, provide a copy of the Resources section at the end of this chapter. This list includes information about all the types of resources that are commonly available for people with dementia and their care partners. When addressing issues specifically associated with mild, moderate, or advanced dementia, provide copies of the resource lists in Chapter 7, Nursing Interventions for Early-Stage Dementia, Chapter 8, Moderate-Stage Dementia, and Chapter 9, Caring for the Person With Advanced Dementia.

In the words of a caregiver:

> There were many times I did not know what to do. . . . I would call the 800 help number and I would say "I do not know what to do. She is freaking—I am freaking out—and I do not know how to handle this." There was always somebody there to answer the phone. (Truglio-Londrigan & Slyer, 2019, p. 258)

RESOURCES FOR ASSISTANCE WITH CARE

Respite care refers to any service whose primary purpose is to relieve caregivers from their usual responsibilities for a short term. The typical recipient of respite care is a person with dementia who lives with a spouse, family member, or other care partner and requires daily or full-time assistance or supervision. Sources of respite care are:

- Adult day care
- Short-term care in a residential facility
- In-home companions or home health aides

Care partners can arrange for respite services when they need time off for work or for personal reasons—including stress reduction—or even for vacations. Nurses caring for people with dementia in acute care or other short-term care settings often are aware of the tremendous stress placed on care partners. In these situations, address the needs of the care partners by asking if they have considered using respite services and introduce this idea as a self-wellness intervention for the care partners. By initiating a discussion of respite care, you may be providing the "permission" that stressed caregivers need to take care of themselves.

Fast Facts

Nurses can suggest that caregivers consider respite services as a self-wellness intervention to reduce stress.

Clinical Snapshot

Mr. U lives with his daughter and has been admitted for uncontrolled diabetes and hypertension. His daughter confides that she is feeling very stressed about being responsible for her father's care as his needs have increased significantly during the past 6 months. Her husband wants her to go with him for 5 days when he is attending a conference in a place they have always wanted to see. You tell her there are many options for short-term care for her father while she is gone and you make a referral for social services.

In the words of the husband of someone with dementia:

It took two years for me to overcome my feelings that I had the primary responsibility to take care of my wife. They had to give me permission to engage this wonderful caregiver. And, that changed my life. I had somebody. (Truglio-Londrigan & Slyer, 2019, p. 260)

ADULT DAY CENTERS

Adult day centers, which are available in most communities, provide structured activities in a group setting for older people with cognitive and functional impairments. Adult day centers typically provide meals, social and recreational activities, and one or more of the following services:

- Transportation
- Medication management
- Assistance with personal care
- Monitoring of health status
- Group outings
- Music and art activities
- Religious services

These programs usually are available on weekdays for up to 8 hours a day; less commonly, some services are available for longer hours and on weekends and holidays. Studies have confirmed that day care programs can improve quality of life for people with dementia as well as their care partners.

RESIDENTIAL CARE FOR PEOPLE WITH DEMENTIA

Although nurses are usually not involved with decisions about residential care for people with dementia, they are responsible for developing discharge plans that provide for safe and appropriate living arrangements. This is especially important when planning care for people with dementia who have medical conditions that require strict adherence to a treatment plan but do not meet the criteria for skilled care, as illustrated in the Clinical Snapshot at the end of this chapter. Also, because traditional nursing homes are often associated with negative images, nurses can encourage care partners to explore the newer models for residential care of people with dementia.

Newer Models for Residential Care

Many nursing homes have developed **specialized dementia, or memory support, programs**. A typical dementia program in a nursing facility is a separate unit with controlled access and exit so that the residents cannot leave without supervision. These programs are suitable for people with moderate-to-advanced dementia who have some degree of mobility and can participate in group activities. Similar to other nursing home units in many ways, the activities are developed specifically for people with dementia, and all staff members are trained for dementia care.

Another recent development for residential care is a **dementia assisted living facility**, which is most appropriate for people with mild-to-moderate dementia. These facilities are either free standing or a part of a long-term care facility or continuing care community. Sometimes, they are separate units with controlled access within a larger assisted living facility. A typical dementia assisted living facility is designed with 16 or more individual rooms in a square around a courtyard to permit residents safe access to the entire indoor and outdoor space. Shared space usually includes sitting rooms, a kitchen area, and large activity rooms. Residents participate in group activities, eat their meals in a dining room, and have assistance with activities of daily living.

Small group homes, which have been available for decades with varying levels of state and federal regulation, are another option for residential care of people with dementia. The Green House Project is a nonprofit organization that began in 2003, as an alternative to traditional nursing facilities and is approved for Medicare and Medicaid funds. These "small-house nursing homes" provide personalized care in intentional communities of 7 to 10 older adults with chronic conditions, including mild dementia. There were more than 150 Green House Project homes in 33 states in 2019, with the expectation that this project will continue to expand.

HOSPICE AND PALLIATIVE CARE SERVICES

Hospice and palliative care services are increasingly available for people with dementia in any setting, with the primary goal of providing support, comfort, and symptom management during the course of progressive illnesses such as dementia. Medicare and other health insurance programs cover both types of care, with the following differences in criteria for hospice or palliative care:

- Hospice services can be initiated when the life expectancy for the person is less than 6 months, whereas palliative care services can be initiated for symptom management at any time during the course of dementia.
- Palliative dementia care services address issues such as the following: pain; loss of appetite; weakness; fatigue; anxiety; depression; sleep disturbances; behavioral changes; and social, emotional, psychological, and spiritual support to the individual and care partners.
- Hospice dementia care addresses these same issues as well as end-of-life concerns.

Nurses are in key positions to identify the need, teach about the benefits, and suggest that care partners explore options for these services.
These services are appropriate for people with advanced dementia,
even without other medical conditions, and for people with moderate
dementia who also have other serious conditions. For example, people
with advanced dementia may be admitted to the hospital for aspiration
pneumonia because of dysphagia. These situations typically involve
the placement of a nasogastric tube and a decision about long-term
ways to provide nutrition. If a decision is made to forego a long-term
feeding tube, hospice or palliative care services may be beneficial for
assisting with comfort feeding and other related issues.

Fast Facts

A wide range of new residential models, along with hospice and
palliative care services, addresses dementia-related issues and
provides social, emotional, psychological, and spiritual support to
people with dementia and their care partners.

⟳ Clinical Snapshot: Discharge Plans for a Patient With Congestive Heart Failure

During the past 6 months, Sophie Walker has been admitted
three times to the medical floor where you work for exacerbation
of congestive heart failure. After the first admission, she received
care in a skilled nursing facility for 10 days and then insisted on
returning to her own home to manage her care independently.
When Sophie's condition worsened after a month, she was read-
mitted to the hospital and then discharged home after 3 days.
She qualified for skilled nursing services from the visiting nurse
association and remained stable for 2 months. When she was
admitted the third time, she had not been taking her medications
correctly and the mental status assessment indicated progressive
memory impairment and other cognitive limitations. Because she
attended social and nutrition programs at the local senior center, she was not homebound and no longer qualified for skilled
nursing services to assist with her medical management at home.
Sophie's doctor indicated that the repeated hospitalizations
could be prevented if her medications were managed appropriately and her medical condition monitored closely. When Sophie's
daughter visits, she confides that she is very frustrated because

(continued)

(continued)

she is the only family member involved with her mother's care and she lives 300 miles away and works full time. You give her the list of the Resources from this chapter and suggest she contact a geriatric care manager to assist her with developing a plan. You also provide information about dementia assisted living facilities and suggest she explore options with her mother.

Reference

Truglio-Londrigan, M., & Slyer, J. (2019). Caregiver decisions along the Alzheimer's disease trajectory. *Geriatric Nursing, 40*, 257–263. doi:10.1016/j.gerinurse.2018.10.015

RESOURCES

Alzheimer's Association
https://www.alz.org

- "One-stop shopping" for information about support and education groups and all resources discussed in this chapter
- 24-7 helpline for advice and information about all types of resources: 800-272-3900

Family Caregiver Alliance
https://www.caregiver.org

- Information about dementia, stresses of caregiving, and resources for family caregivers

HelpGuide
https://www.helpguide.org

- Information about dementia and caregiver issues
- Links to resources, including respite, adult day care, and hospice and palliative care

National Association of Professional Geriatric Care Managers
https://www.caremanager.org

- Information about geriatric care managers
- Directory of geriatric care managers by zip code

National Eldercare Locator
https://www.eldercare.gov

- Information specialists available Monday to Friday 9 a.m. to 8 p.m. ET at 800-677-1116 or online

National Hospice and Palliative Care Organization
https://www.nhpco.org

- Information about hospice and palliative care for dementia

Index

abuse, alcohol, 18–19, 162
accurate patient information,
 obtaining, 120–121
 cultural considerations, 121–122
ACE. *See* Acute Care for the Elderly
 units
acetaminophen (Tylenol), 153
activities of daily living (ADL), 128
activity. *See also* daily activities,
 issues related to
 inadequate physical activity, and
  fall risks, 141
 level, and advanced dementia,
  86
 self-care activities, 155
Acute Care for the Elderly (ACE)
 units, 123
ADL. *See* activities of daily living
adult day centers, 178
adult protective service laws,
 164–165
advanced dementia, 10–11, 13
 care for comfort, 92
 characteristics of, 86–87
 communication issues during,
  57–58
 conditions that increase fall
  risks in, 138
 cultural considerations, 91–92
 emotional needs during,
  99–100

nutrition, challenges related to,
 89–90
supportive and end-of-life care,
 90–91
treatment goals, 87–88
advanced directives, 172–174
aggressive behaviors, 109–111
 nursing actions to address,
  110–111
akathisia, 144
alcohol abuse, 162
 and mental changes, 18–19
altered perception of reality,
 108–109
Alzheimer's Association, 13, 46,
 73, 75, 81, 84, 115, 126, 145, 171,
 176, 181
Alzheimer's disease, 5, 6, 8, 99
American Geriatrics Society, 21–22
analgesics, 152
 opioid, 153
 topical, 153
antianxiety agents, 44
anticholinergic medications, 28
 and mental changes, 18
anticonvulsants, 153
antidepressants, 101, 153
antipsychotics, 44, 113, 114
assisted living facility, 179
attention, redirection of, 108
auditory hallucinations, 108

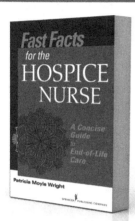
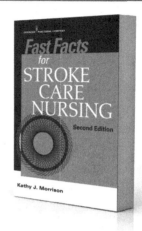
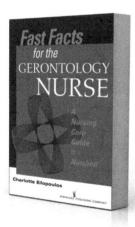
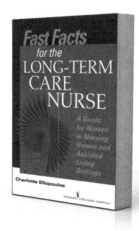

Printed in the United States
by Baker & Taylor Publisher Services